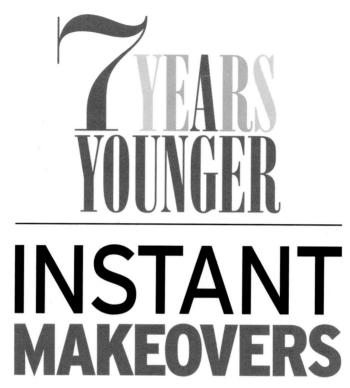

7 YEARS YOUNGER

INSTANT MAKEOVERS

The Quick & Easy Anti-Aging Plan for Beautiful Skin, Hair, Mind & Body

**BY THE EDITORS OF
WOMAN'S DAY MAGAZINE**

Hearst Editions
An imprint of Hearst Magazines

Contents

See It, Believe It!

Meet our 7 Years Younger Panelists, and find out which mini-makeovers worked for them.

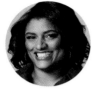

Mandy Roberson, 42,
Restore Dry, Damaged Hair, p. 20

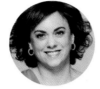

Fern Richter, 45,
Add Fullness to Hair,
p. 30

Gabrielle Kennedy, 36,
Add Volume to Hair,
p. 34

Jacqueline DeMuro, 48,
Go Gray the Right Way,
p. 40

Mary Ellen Sanchez, 56,
Give Hair Shape,
p. 50

Jade Dillman, 42,
Bring Bounce to Hair,
p. 54

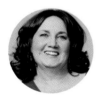

Eileen Wharton, 50,
Get an Instant Face Lift, p. 64

Tessa Jean, 37,
Brighten a Dull Complexion, p. 68

Silvia Robles, 42,
Perk Up Tired Eyes,
p. 102

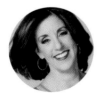

Estelle Schmones, 64,
Play Up Eyes,
p. 110

Diane Durando, 44,
Plump Lips,
p. 132

Jackie Plant, 52,
Revitalize Damaged Skin, p. 158

Acknowledgments

Most of us don't have a stylist, hairdresser, personal trainer and nutritionist to keep aging at bay. All of that takes time, and really, who has time in abundance these days?

So the editors of *Woman's Day* created this book, the third in the best-selling *7 Years Younger* series, that gives you quick tools to help you look and feel younger: easy tweaks like the best way to apply mascara so it doesn't look like a clumpy mess (p. 117), the benefits of taking a "hair vacation" (p. 16) and how to make critical changes to your sleep routine—hello, thinner pillow! (p. 281)—to ensure better rest.

The driving force behind *7 Years Younger Instant Makeovers* is WD's talented and indefatigable executive editor Annemarie Conte, who headed up an army of editors, photographers, designers, beauty and style experts, and many, many other contributors. Huge kudos go to Annemarie as well as Kim Tranell, who brought this subject to life with her excellent reporting and writing, and WD beauty editor Melissa Matthews Brown, whose depth of expertise in the beauty field gave our anti-aging advice both science and practicality. Health director Abigail Cuffey, food and nutrition director Kate Merker, senior associate food editor Yasmin Sabir, style editor Donna Duarte-Ladd and assistant style and beauty editor Maureen Sheen also contributed their expertise. Our ace copy editor Lauren Spencer kept everyone in line grammatically, assistant features editor Anna Dysinger organized us all with her usual calm efficiency, and managing editor Sue Kakstys kept us on track and on budget.

The amazing art team, led by *Woman's Day* creative director Sara Williams, carried out our vision of a pretty (and useful) book. Thanks go to photo director Stephanie Kim and photo researcher Sara Neumann, chief designer Andrea Brake Lukeman and photographer Shannon Greer.

Because this book focuses so much on beauty, we called in the pros. Big thanks to Laura Geller, Roy Liu and Andrea Coombs Angrilla for Laura Geller Beauty; makeup artist Sue Pike; Nunzio Saviano, hairstylist Lauren Thompson and colorist John Whelan and Stephanie Brown for the Nunzio Saviano Salon; Kyle White and team from the Oscar Blandi Salon; and clothing stylist Maria-Stefania Vavylopoulou.

We would be nowhere without publisher Jacqueline Deval and creative director of content extensions Mark Gompertz, whose vision underlies all our efforts, along with their team, marketing director Tom McLean, product manager TJ Mancini and assistant managing editor Kim Jaso. Thanks, too, to my fellow editors-in-chief, Jane Francisco of *Good Housekeeping*, Rachel Barrett of *Country Living*, and Jill Herzig of *Redbook*.

The support of the executive team at Hearst has been critical to *7 Years Younger*, and I'd like to acknowledge David Carey, president, Hearst Magazines; Michael Clinton, president, marketing & publishing director; John Loughlin, executive vice president & general manager; Ellen Levine, editorial director; and Alexandra Carlin, vice president of public relations.

Finally, thank you to our makeover panelists. They were beautiful at the start, and even more so now.

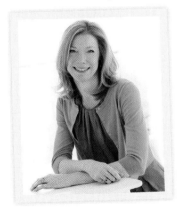

Enjoy every page of *7 Years Younger Instant Makeovers*. Try them, share them with your friends, and reap the benefits.

Susan

Susan Spencer
Editor-in-Chief, Woman's Day
susan@womansday.com

Introduction: Take Years Off — in Minutes!

There's a confusing contradiction that happens as you get older. Some days, you look in the mirror—focused on that one fine line you *swear* wasn't there yesterday—and become frustrated. It's like your appearance doesn't represent how young and vibrant you feel on the inside. Other days, though, you actually feel your age—maybe even older. And you worry: Will all that internal chaos start to show on the outside? You suspect it will, but even so, you try to dismiss these concerns—because you're convinced there's no way you'll ever find the time to actually do something about them.

Until now. Through the research done for *7 Years Younger* and the *7 Years Younger Anti-Aging Diet*, we know that turning back the clock is possible. With the right combination of smart hair and skincare, good nutrition, consistent exercise, sufficient sleep and strategic stress relief, you *can* look and feel younger. And while we stand by the promise that we made in *7 Years Younger*—that our comprehensive beauty, diet and fitness program will deliver results in just seven weeks—we also understand that not every woman has the time or desire to overhaul her entire life. That's where this mini-makeover manual steps in.

Anti-Aging Advice That's Backed by Experts

When we talked to readers, they told us they wanted a handbook for looking younger *now*, full of super-fast tools, tactics and tricks to solve their biggest beauty and skin problems or to help them make the lifestyle changes needed for weight loss and stress relief. So we combed through the anti-aging research and grilled the very best experts (learn more about them in our 7 Years Younger Expert Directory, p. 316) to come up with bite-size advice, all packaged into easy makeovers. We also used the savvy staff at *Woman's Day* and the Good Housekeeping Research Institute, which has a deep database of anti-aging product tests—so that we could be sure our recommendations give you the best bang for your buck. We also drew on the anti-aging experts at *Redbook* magazine.

Finally—and perhaps most important—we asked our 7 Years Younger Panel, made up of 12 *Woman's Day* readers ranging in age from 36 to 64, to test out our advice. Through their feedback, we know that we're making the best recommendations for both in-the-moment fixes *and* long-term solutions that fit seamlessly into your daily routine and your budget. (You can read all about the 7 Years Younger Panel, and see their before/after photos, starting on page 20.)

How to Use This Book

Reading this mini-makeover manual from cover to cover will definitely help to demystify the aging process, but don't be overwhelmed—it certainly isn't recommended that you try *all* of its advice. Instead, look at this as your ultimate beauty and health handbook to consult any time a problem pops up ("why am I having trouble falling asleep?") or whenever you want the confidence that comes from giving your skin or hair a little extra attention ("it's about time I tackle those dark undereye circles!"). To help you do this easily and efficiently, the advice is divided into two sections:

CHAPTERS 1 TO 5

- Learn the hairstyling secrets, makeup tricks and skincare solutions. And many of the Mini-Makeovers are two-in-one: You'll get a quick fix (how the right lipstick can make your teeth look brighter) as well as a lasting solution (an affordable whitening treatment).

CHAPTERS 6 TO 9

- Poor sleep, high stress levels, not enough exercise, the wrong foods—each of these factors can affect your health, your appearance *and* your energy levels in ways you may never have realized. Luckily, though, the Mini-Makeovers in this section make it easy to identify your problem areas—and provide easy, actionable ways to rehab your habits for ultimate health and happiness.

7 Years Younger's Biggest Benefit

We learned quite a bit from the readers who tested our advice. A predominant theme that came up in almost every single conversation, and one that we think is worth mentioning up front, is this: These busy women were all pleasantly surprised by how much joy and confidence they gained from building just a *little* more "me" time into their day—whether they were using that extra 2 minutes for meditation or makeup. "If you just take the time to put yourself higher on the priority list, you can learn little things to do daily that change your appearance *and* outlook," said Silvia Robles, 42 (p. 102). Fellow panelist Jade Dillman, 42, agreed (p. 54): "Knowing there are things I can do to feel great about myself is one thing, but knowing that I can do it myself is what really matters."

7 Years Younger Anti-Aging Resources

Free Stuff

- Receive our weekly anti-aging newsletter at *7yearsyounger.com/ newsletter*

- Download our anti-aging reports, filled with helpful, doable tips:

  - 40 Best Anti-Aging Beauty Secrets at *7yearsyounger.com/ antiagingsecrets*

  - Best Anti-Aging Makeup at *7yearsyounger.com/makeup*

  - Eat to Look and Feel Younger at *7yearsyounger.com/eattolookyoung*

  - 50 Ways to Stress Less & Live Longer at *7yearsyounger.com/ stressless*

Shopping

- To find the top rated anti-aging beauty products mentioned in this book, visit *7yearsyounger.com/shop*

- To buy a copy of *The New York Times* best seller *7 Years Younger: The Revolutionary 7-Week Anti-Aging Plan*, go to *7yearsyounger.com/book*

- To buy a copy of the *7 Years Younger Anti-Aging Breakthrough Diet* and the *7 Years Younger Anti-Aging Breakthrough Diet Workbook*, go to *7yearsyounger.com/diet*

- To get more anti-aging, health and diet news, subscribe to *Woman's Day* at *7yysub.womansday.com*, to *Good Housekeeping* at *7yysub. goodhousekeeping.com*, and to *Redbook* at *7yysub.redbookmag.com*

Social

- Want to be a test panelist for a future 7 Years Younger plan? Sign up at *7yearsyounger.com/panelist* to be considered

- Like us on *facebook.com/7yearsyounger*

- Follow us on Twitter *@7yearsyounger*

- Follow us on *pinterest.com/7yearsyounger*

Help Your Hair

1

How to deal with hair that's dry, damaged or thinning. Plus, going gray the right way—and youth-boosting cuts, colors and styles.

66A woman who cuts her hair is about to change her life." *- Coco Chanel*

There's a good chance you've spent more than a few mornings in the bathroom, frustrated that your hair won't do what it used to. It's almost as if your hair has suddenly developed a completely different personality. What's going on? "Aging-related shifts in hair color and texture are universal," says New York City dermatologist Francesca Fusco, MD, who specializes in hair and scalp health. "Genetics play a role, as does how you take care of your hair."

To demystify the hair-aging process, it helps to understand what's happening. Simply put, hair follicles get smaller over time, so the hairs they produce become thinner. This causes limpness and lack of volume. The scalp also produces less oil, which zaps moisture, manageability and shine. What's more, years of styling with heat, harsh dyes and chemical relaxers make hair less healthy and more prone to breakage and frizz. "The good news is, you *can* restore the hair and prevent more damage," says Kevin Mancuso, celebrity hairstylist and creative director for Nexxus. "You just need to change the way you care for it." In the chapter ahead, learn how to bring back shine, softness and bounce to your hair, while learning how it can take years off your appearance.

MINI-MAKEOVER #1
Restore Softness and Shine

FIX IT FAST

Deeply Condition and Add Gloss

If you're battling dry, brittle locks, a few tweaks to the way you wash and style your hair can give it new life—almost instantly! Here's exactly how to rehab your routine, starting with your very next shower:

1 **Check your shampoo.** Don't use a clarifying shampoo more than once a week (or more than once or twice a month for textured hair types, which are naturally drier). Because these cleansers are formulated to remove product buildup, they strip hair's natural oils, too. Instead, try a shampoo for dry hair, which contains extra moisturizing agents, or an aging-related formula (See: Ask the Experts, p. 14), which hydrates and adds shine to regular or color-treated hair without over-softening. **TRY: Nexxus Youth Renewal Rejuvenating Shampoo** ($13; *7yearsyounger.com/shop*).

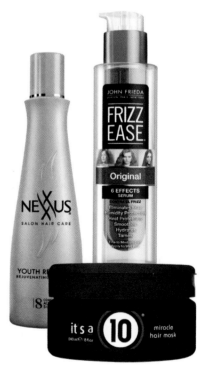

2 **Deeply condition.** Take your regular conditioner and spread it on from scalp to tips, letting it soak in for 2 to 3 minutes before rinsing. Then, once a week, apply a hydrating hair mask. "Look for deeply hydrating ingredients like sunflower

QUICK TIP

Repair dry, damaged hair with avocado. The healthy fats in this fruit can help strengthen and nourish hair that's broken due to sun and styling. Just mash up a ripe avocado and apply it as a prewash treatment. Leave in for 30 minutes, then rinse and shampoo. **Cost: $1.25**

oil, avocado oil or almond oil," says Dr. Fusco. **TRY: It's a 10 Miracle Hair Mask** ($21; *7yearsyounger.com/shop*).

3 **Give it polish.** At the end of your shower, turn the nozzle and rinse your hair out with cold water for 5 to 10 seconds. (This closes the cuticle, for more shine.) Hair should feel noticeably softer and look shinier once dry, but you can add extra sleekness to straight or wavy hair with a lightweight finishing product. Rub a tiny drop (a little goes a long way) between hands, then smooth over hair from part to ends. **TRY: John Frieda Frizz-Ease Original Six Effects Serum** ($8; *7yearsyounger.com/shop*).

ASK THE EXPERTS *What Are Anti-Aging Hair Products?*

High-tech ingredients are no longer limited to face lotions. A slew of anti-agers, like niacinamide and caffeine, are debuting in hair products, says Jeni Thomas, PhD, a scientist at Proctor & Gamble, which developed the Pantene Age Defy line. Mancuso, who worked on Nexxus's Youth Renewal line, adds that most anti-aging products are carefully formulated to balance the many issues you may face as you age. "Maybe it used to be that your hair was just dry, so you could pick a shampoo and conditioner for dry hair," Mancuso says. "But as you get older your hair may be dry, thinning, limp and colored." Anti-aging products attempt to do it all.

FIX IT SO IT LASTS

Try a Leave-in Treatment or Glaze

Repairing hair that's dry and dull can be tricky, says Mancuso—you want to give it sleekness and moisture, but too many women go too far, making strands slippery and lifeless. So start with the simple changes from the previous pages, and if you still feel like you need more moisture, shine or manageability, consider these options:

For more strengthening and softening:

- **Use a leave-in treatment.** Hair serums, lotions and creams designed for aging hair provide a mix of ingredients that strengthen strands, restore moisture, add shine, and prevent breakage. (Warning: They're potent, so start by adding just a drop to damp hair so it doesn't get greasy.) **TRY: Alterna Haircare Caviar Anti-aging Omega + Nourishing Oil** ($38; *sephora.com*).

- **To restore softness and moisture**, coarse curls or textured hair can also benefit from a DIY Steamer treatment (See Savings Tip: p. 29).

If you're satisfied with softness but crave more shine:

- **Get a gloss or glaze.** These salon treatments (on average $20 to $50, depending on location, but sometimes free with salon color service) are to your hair what a topcoat is to your nails, says Dr. Fusco. They deposit either a clear or pigmented coating over the length of your strands to smooth the cuticle and increase sheen, and they last for up to four weeks. Ask for one at your next cut or color appointment, or use an at-home product once a week after you shampoo and condition. **TRY: Rita Hazan Ultimate Shine Color Gloss in Clear** ($15; *7yearsyounger.com/shop*).

HABIT REHAB
Protect Brittle Hair from Breakage

Dry, dull hair that's lacking moisture is more prone to damage—but a few simple tweaks to your styling routine can keep strands safe.

1. Get regular trims. A cut every six to eight weeks will lob off damaged ends that weaken strands. (Even if you wear your hair natural, this is key, says Toni Garcia-Jackson, a hairstylist in Wilmington, Delaware, because split ends are inevitable, even if you aren't styling with heat or chemicals.)

2. Update your brush. "Older brushes often have missing or broken bristles that snag hair and cause breakage," says Mancuso. For a brush that won't pull or put hair under stress as you're styling, try one with natural bristles or flexible synthetic bristles. **TRY: The Wet Brush** ($14; *thewetbrush.com*).

3. Prep for heat. Before you blow-dry or curl, always apply a hydrating heat protection spray to damp hair. They're formulated with conditioning ingredients, like glycerin, to coat strands and help combat the drying effects of heated styling tools. **TRY: Herbal Essences Set Me Up Heat Protection Spray** ($5.99; *7yearsyounger.com/shop*).

4. Turn down the temp—and be gentle. Keep curling irons and flat irons on low settings, and lightly twirl or squeeze hair. "You're better off doing a second pass with your flat iron than applying lots of pressure and heat all at once," says Mancuso.

5. Switch to a better blow dryer. The next time your dryer dies, replace it with one that's ionic and ceramic. It shortens drying time while reducing heat damage. **TRY: Remington T-Studio Silk Ceramic Blow Dryer** ($32.96; *7yearsyounger.com/shop*).

6. Give hair a holiday. Damaged strands need a break, so take advantage of lazy weekend days to let hair rest and repair, says Dr. Fusco—no dryer, no flat iron, no product. Even one day a week without heat will work wonders!

SAVINGS TIP! **Use tea as a DIY gloss.** Brew two tea bags in 2 cups of hot water (chamomile for blondes, rooibos for redheads and black for brunettes), let it cool, then apply the liquid as a final rinse at the end of your shower. The tea mixture closes the cuticle, which smooths hair and adds polish, while also boosting color or neutralizing brassiness, says Philip Pelusi, CEO of Tela Beauty Organics. **Cost per treatment: 40¢**

MINI-MAKEOVER #2
Bring Back Body and Bounce

Why is your hair looking a little lifeless lately, even after blow-drying? The growth cycle of your hair follicles slows down every year, resulting in fewer strands, and those fewer strands are also getting finer. In addition to these changes, which are programmed into your DNA (well-intentioned styling and overuse of conditioning treatments—meant to combat age-related dryness and dullness—can take their toll). "It's what I call over-softening," says Mancuso. "Too much conditioning or polishing can reduce the volume and make hair slippery and flat."

FIX IT FAST **Style to Boost Body**

When faced with limp locks, many women attempt to add body by curling or styling the ends, "but all that does is weigh the hair down, so it collapses," says Rodney Cutler, a celebrity hairstylist. "If you want to add volume, it has to come from the roots down." These tips from the pros will help tweak your styling routine so hair has lift and movement:

1 **Bump up the allover volume.** Start with a volumizing product, like mousse. Work a golf-ball-size sphere through clean, wet hair from roots to tips. **TRY: L'Oréal Advanced Hairstyle BOOST It Volume Inject Mousse** ($4.99; at drugstores).

2 **Lift from the roots.** This step is crucial: Pick up sections of hair along the part and crown, and spray roots directly with a booster (most can be used on damp or dry hair). **TRY: John Frieda Luxurious Volume Root Booster Blow Dry Lotion** ($7; *7yearsyounger.com/shop*).

3 **Re-think your blow-dry.** To boost body, flip your head over first, until hair is about 85 percent dry. (Those with cropped cuts can stay upright.) "The key is that you get your fingers in there at the roots and tousle it around," says Mancuso. You can still add sleekness with a paddle brush or curl ends under with a round brush at the very end, and for extra oomph, roll back three Velcro rollers in the front section (left, middle and right) for 10 to 15 minutes. TIP: Let rollers set while you apply your makeup or eat breakfast.

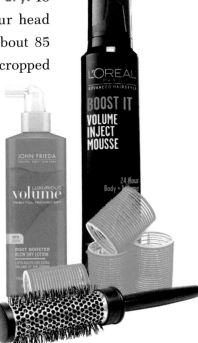

Re-Do Your Regimen

The wrong shampoos, conditioners and stylers might deposit too much shine and slipperiness on fine hair, but the right ones can plump strands and boost body. Here's how to switch up your products and banish buildup that makes hair fall flat:

- **Every day:** To cut down on slick residue, look for shampoos and conditioners that are free of heavy silicones, or use products for aging hair. Many are designed to temporarily increase the diameter of each hair shaft for more overall volume. **TRY: Bosley Professional Strength Bos Defense Nourishing Shampoo** ($22.50; *7yearsyounger.com/shop*).

- **Once a week:** Use a clarifying shampoo, which removes product residue. **TRY: Aubrey Green Tea Shampoo** ($10.95; *7yearsyounger.com/shop*). (One note: Because these shampoos can be extra-drying, women with textured hair, which is naturally drier, should use them no more than once or twice a month.) Then, to deeply condition—even fine hair needs more moisture—you may want to avoid heavy oils, and go for a lighter formulation, which hydrates hair without weighing it down. Apply from mid-shaft to ends, where hair is driest. **TRY: Nexxus Hydra-Light Weightless Moisture Leave-In Conditioning Foam** ($12; *7yearsyounger.com/shop*).

> **QUICK TIP**
>
> **Does your relaxed hair lack body?** Consider a texturizer instead, says Garcia-Jackson. "If a relaxer is like a well-done steak, a texturizer would be medium-rare," she explains. "It stays on for less time and leaves some of your natural curl, which will create the illusion of thicker, fuller hair as you get older."

SAVINGS TIP! **Try this DIY clarifying rinse.** To nix product buildup and restore shine and bounce, combine $1/2$ cup of apple cider vinegar with the juice from a quarter of a lemon. Work the mix through dry hair before you shampoo. **Cost per recipe: 30¢**

7 YEARS YOUNGER MAKEOVER
The Problem: Damaged Hair

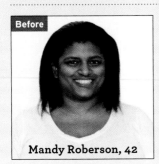

Before

Mandy Roberson, 42

Mandy had been coloring and relaxing her own hair for years to save time and money. She skipped deep conditioners and frequent trims needed to keep chemically treated hair healthy, so her hair is weak and brittle. "My mom has Alzheimer's disease, my dad suffered a stroke, and I'm also raising my 3-year-old daughter," says Mandy. "Honestly, I'm good at taking care of everybody except me." As an entrepreneur, she is constantly going to meetings and networking and would like her hair to be healthy, but also stylish.

THE FIX:

- **More Color in Her Hair:** Mandy's skin and hair were all one tone, so Kyle White, a colorist at Oscar Blandi Salon in New York City, warmed her up and covered grays with a rich chestnut brown. Then he added a few toffee highlights for dimension and to boost shine. (See: Make It Multi-Dimensional, p. 43.)
- **Protect Hair from Heated Styling Tools:** Mandy's planning to prep her hair with **a heat protectant spray** before she blow-dries. White also suggests she invest in a good blow dryer, one that will minimize damage. (See: Habit Rehab, p. 16.)

FINISHING TOUCHES

1. Groom Brows: Thinning out Mandy's brows slightly and creating an arch mid-brow helps lift eyes and frames her face.

2. Always Apply Blush: A little cheek color helps to emphasize her beautiful bone structure. This rosy pink hue gives Mandy a youth boost.

3. Wear a Bright Top: Adding a pop of color close to her face helps light up her complexion and evoke confidence.

66
Now I see what a little TLC for my hair can do for me."
—Mandy

MINI-MAKEOVER #3
Smooth Out Frizzy, Wiry Hair

 Give Hair a Blowout

Because wiriness is likely caused by little bends to the hair's cuticle (that's the outer layer of each strand), blow-drying is key. The heat straightens the kinks, while also taming flyways. Follow this quick tutorial for a smoother, sleeker finish:

1 **Prep with product.** Apply a blow-dry lotion to damp hair to build volume and protect hair from the dryer's heat. Run the dryer over your head until your hair is 50 percent dry. **TRY: Blow Ready Set Blow Express Blow Dry Lotion** ($21; *7yearsyounger.com/shop*).

TRY: Your Best Frizz-Fighters

These three smoothing, shine-enhancing stylers came out on top in Good Housekeeping Research Institute tests:

- **OVERALL WINNER: Joico K-PAK Protect & Shine Serum** ($14.30; *7yearsyounger.com/shop*) Testers liked the lightweight texture, which left their hair soft, not greasy.

- **TESTERS' CHOICE: Garnier Fructis Sleek & Shine Anti-Frizz Serum** ($6; at drugstores) An impressive 91 percent of testers said they'd continue using this styler, crediting its frizz-taming and shine-enhancing abilities.

- **BUDGET BUY: Suave Professionals Sleek Anti-Frizz Cream** ($3; *drugstore.com*) This bargain was the only winning cream, and many testers said they liked using a cream product better than a serum.

2 **Straighten and smooth.** Hold your dryer up high and point it down, so that the stream of heat travels along the shaft, from roots to end. (This is critical, as it closes the cuticle and prevents frizz.)

- **For hair chin-length or longer:** Divide hair into three sections, one in front and two in back. Then, further divide each section into three smaller ones. Run a round brush through each section from root to end as you blow-dry it straight.

- **For short hair:** Use a flat brush (boar-hair bristles are best to tame your new texture), and move the blow-dryer with the brush, using the air to direct the hair in the direction you want it to go.

3 **Add polish.** Shine enhancers are formulated to smooth the cuticle, so apply one on dry hair as a final styling step. Rub product between hands first, then smooth hands over hair from roots to ends. (See: Your Best Frizz-Fighters, p. 22.)

Do a Smoothing Treatment

Age-related dryness can contribute to texture changes and intensify frizz, so it's crucial to deep condition and moisturize. (See: Restore Softness and Shine, p. 13.) From there, use a keratin treatment, says hairstylist Jet Rhys. At a salon, these services are pricey (about $200, three times a year), but now the same ingredients are in drugstore products for a fraction of the cost. **TRY: OGX Express Ever Straight Brazilian Keratin Therapy 14 Day Smoothing Treatment** ($4.24; *7yearsyounger.com/shop*). Our testers liked that this product was simple to apply: Spray onto 80 percent dry hair and expect "smoothness for days."

Tips for Transitioning Relaxed Hair

Thinking about going natural? Here's what you need to know about smoothing the transition from relaxed to textured hair:

1. Pick the right style. Having stronger, natural hair coming in at the roots and weaker, relaxed hair growing out on the bottom is a recipe for breakage, says Garcia-Jackson. So choose a style that blends the two textures with minimal stress to the hair, like roller sets or twist-outs.

2. Make sure your scalp is healthy. Using a shampoo or scalp treatment with an exfoliating ingredient, like salicylic acid, unclogs pores and gets rid of product build-up that suffocates follicles. This helps textured hair grow in fuller and healthier.

3. Treat both textures. Moisturizing with hair masks will decrease splitting and shedding, but you may need to mix products into a "cocktail" to target the needs of both textures. Talk to your hairstylist about a deep conditioning regimen that's right for you.

4. Get regular trims. Even if you're no longer chemically treating hair or heat styling, you still need a cut every six to eight weeks. "Splitting occurs naturally. Your goal is to gain length, and trims keep hair growing healthy and strong," says Garcia-Jackson.

5. Be gentle. The "line of demarcation"—where your natural hair meets your relaxed hair—is incredibly fragile. So after applying your leave-in conditioner, section your hair, then detangle it carefully with your fingers, starting at the ends and working up to the roots. Avoid heat whenever possible.

6. Work with a pro. "Your new hair is not going to behave like your relaxed hair, and that's OK," says Garcia-Jackson. Finding a stylist who knows how to manage your new texture—and who can teach you about your curl type—is key to feeling confident while you wait it out.

MINI-MAKEOVER #4
Define Your Curls

As you age, you may notice that your curls are more difficult to manage. Just as straight hair can get kinky, curly hair can change in texture, too. Some ringlets may look a bit frizzier, while others lose some of their structure and integrity. "Because of the miniaturization of the hair shaft, each hair is becoming thinner, and its diameter can be different from root to end," says Mancuso. "Your curl may become more oval at the bottom, and rounder closer to the scalp."

> **QUICK TIP**
> **Avoid an unflattering cut.** With an extremely wiry texture, you may want to rethink your short 'do. A cut that's mid-neck to collarbone-grazing works best, says Rhys. "The shorter you go, the more hair expands," she says, "and poofiness looks aging."

 FIX IT FAST   ### Smooth and Shape Curls

Soft, non-crunchy curls are instantly de-aging, so less styling is more flattering—and defining your curls starts in the shower. Follow this tutorial to set yourself up for a frizz-free look:

1 **Cleanse carefully.** Curly hair is drier than straight hair, so if you're not already, make sure you shampoo less frequently and use a sulfate-free formula to preserve more of your natural oils. **TRY: DevaCurl No-Poo or Low-Poo** ($19; *sephora.com*). To keep curls looking fresh in between, you can use a co-wash, which gently cleanses and hydrates at the same time. Fine hair can be cleansed every other day, while women with coarser or more textured hair should stick to twice a week. **TRY: SheaMoisture Coconut & Hibiscus Co-Wash Conditioning Cleanser** ($18.49; *7yearsyounger.com/shop*).

2 **Condition.** Curls need a lot of moisture, so apply an ultramoisturizing conditioner all over hair; then, gently work it through with a wide-tooth comb or your fingers. Let it penetrate for 2 to 3 minutes, then rinse. **TRY: As I Am Hydration Elation Intensive Conditioner** ($15.49; *7yearsyounger.com/shop*).

3 **Set it—and forget it.** Hands off that towel! Before you even get out of the shower, apply a leave-in product formulated to enhance natural curls. Put it on soaking wet hair (this locks in moisture), using a wide-tooth comb to evenly distribute from roots to ends (See: Curl Hair Control, *below*). Don't touch hair while you let it dry—this is the number-one cause of frizz.

TRY: Curly Hair Control

A daily leave-in product formulated for naturally curly hair is a must. "These products add definition, enhance shine and fight frizz," explains Tippi Shorter, a celebrity hairstylist who has worked with Beyoncé and Jennifer Hudson, and who is also Aveda's Global Artistic Director for textured hair. You might already be using one, but make sure it matches your hair's thickness and texture—as well as your curl type. (Otherwise, it could compromise the quality of your curls.) Your stylist can help, but here are some general rules:

- **If your hair is fine and soft to the touch:** You'll do well with a leave-in serum treatment that seals the cuticle and intensifies the curl, says Shorter. Apply daily to damp hair and comb through with a wide-tooth comb or fingers for complete coverage. **TRY: Aveda Be-Curly Style-Prep** ($22; *7yearsyounger.com/shop*) **or Redken Curvaceous Full Swirl** ($16.49; *7yearsyounger.com/shop*).

- **For thicker textures:** Coarser hair needs a heavier leave-in product to fight frizz, so look for gels or creams, says Shorter. **TRY: Carol's Daughter Healthy Hair Butter** ($15; *7yearsyounger.com/shop*).

FIX IT SO IT LASTS

Deep-Condition Curls and Add Gloss

According to Shorter, restoring softness and shine are key in managing frizzy curls. Here's how she suggests you do it:

1 **Use a Deep Treatment** Shorter recommends at-home masks, which detangle curls while adding moisture. Look for *hydrating* or *softening* on the label, and women with brittle texture will want natural oils, like coconut, jojoba, avocado or shea butter. **TRY: Carol's Daughter Tui Moisturizing Hair Smoothie** ($19; *7yearsyounger.com/shop*).

2 **Get a Gloss or Glaze** These treatments, which deposit either a clear or pigmented coating over the length of your strands to smooth the cuticle and increase sheen, last up to four weeks. Ask for one at your next cut ($20 to $50).

More Tips for Defining Curls

☑ **On mornings when you don't wash—or to control frizz once hair is dry:** Spray on a curl refresher all over, lifting up sections of hair to make sure it's evenly distributed. This will tame frizz and bring curls, coils or kinks back to life. **TRY: Oiudad Botanical Boost Moisture Infusing & Refreshing Spray** ($16.95; *7yearsyounger.com/shop*).

☑ **To "fake it" with stubborn strands:** If a few ringlets still look zapped, it's OK to twirl hair around a small ⅜-inch curling iron to add shape once in a while. Just be sure to use a low setting and a heat-protectant spray first, so you won't damage hair long-term. **TRY: Hot Tools Professional Spring Curling Iron for Soft, Tight Curls-3/8** ($28.99; *soap.com*)

☑ **To refresh ringlets during the day:** Most curl-refreshers or curl-enhancers are reactivated by water, so simply rewet puffy or frizzy pieces, then twist each one around your finger or a pen to reshape.

QUICK TIP

Switch to a satin pillowcase. To wake up with fresher looking curls on a daily basis, ditch the cotton case, which robs moisture from hair and causes frizz, says Garcia-Jackson. You might also want to pull your hair into a soft, loose ponytail on top of your head before bed—that way curls won't look slept on. (Bonus: A satin pillowcase will also prevent wrinkles!)

MINI-MAKEOVER #5
Create Fuller-Looking Locks

When you grab your hair in your hand, does it feel less hefty than it once did? This aging-related loss of volume is a gradual process programmed into your DNA, says David E. Bank, MD, a dermatologist in Mt. Kisco, New York—and he describes it as having a double-whammy effect. "The average scalp has 100,000 hair follicles," he says. "By the age of 40, some of those follicles will stop producing hair all together, and the rest will sprout strands that are individually thinner and finer than they used to be." What's more, other outside factors (often indirectly related to age)

Why Did My Hair Go From Curly to Straight?

While it's not as common as straight-to-kinky or a loosening of curls, this severe texture change can occur with age, thanks to genetic shifts in your scalp's oil production and the damage that comes from extreme styling, which zaps moisture. "By coloring it with harsh blond dyes or overstyling with flat irons, you can really lose the integrity of your curl," says Rhys. Ringlets may be gone for good, but you might be able to get them back. Your best bet is to stop using all heating elements whatsoever, and attend only to your base color (while eliminating bleach-based highlights). Rhys also recommends a strict regimen of intense at-home masks to restore hair's moisture. (See: Deep-Condition Curls and Add Gloss, p. 27.)

could contribute to shedding too. "From 35 to 55, you're raising a family, you've got kids, work, relationships—maybe you're starting new medications, which could be a factor," says Dr. Bank. "Your stress levels are up, and suddenly the diet is not as good as it used to be either. All of these things lead to hair loss."

FIX IT FAST **Boost Volume and Conceal Sparse Strands**
Try styles and products that will help with thinning.

To Add Overall Volume...

- **Use thickening shampoos and treatments.** Instead of volume-boosting products that just bind fibers together, look for one that contains caffeine or panthenol to increase the diameter of the hairs and bump up volume. **TRY: Pantene AgeDefy Advanced Thickening Treatment** ($13; *7yearsyounger.com/shop*).

- **Get a flattering cut.** "Thin hair should be mid-neck length or shorter and have layers throughout," says Rhys. Style with a root booster, then hold the top sections of your hair straight up as you blow-dry. **TRY: Nexxus Hydra-Light Weightless Moisture Root Lift Mist** ($10; *7yearsyounger.com/shop*).

SAVINGS TIP! **Try a salon softening treatment at home.**
To replicate the steamer yourself, Shorter suggests that after you shampoo and condition apply a couple of drops of eucalyptus or lavender oil to your scalp. Heat a damp hand towel (make sure it's completely wrung out) in the microwave for 20 seconds, put on a plastic shower cap then wrap the steaming towel around the cap (use caution while wrapping since the towel will be hot). Keep it on for 5 to 10 minutes.

7 YEARS YOUNGER MAKEOVER
The Problem: Thin Hair

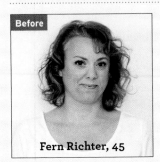

Before

Fern Richter, 45

"My daughter was touching my face, and she asked, 'What are those creases?' I said, 'They're wrinkles!'" says Fern, who has been a 7 Years Younger anti-aging testing panelist for two years. While she's thrilled with the progress she has made by following the program's approach to eating—she's lost 20 pounds so far—Fern was ready to shift her attention to some of her other age-related concerns, like her thin hair and sagging skin.

THE FIX:

- **Lose Length:** Fern was right—her fine hair is thinning, says Nunzio Saviano, owner of the Nunzio Saviano salon in New York City. He removed 2 inches of length, getting rid of her "see-through ends." Then he added face framing layers to give hair more shape. (See: Switch Up the Length, p. 53.)

- **Deepen Hair Color:** Try a warm hue to make hair appear thicker, says John Whelan, a colorist at Saviano's salon. He changed Fern's base to a rich auburn then painted on gold highlights, which also covered the grays that were making her hair look thinner. (See: Pick the Perfect Shade, p. 43.)

FINISHING TOUCHES

1. Fill-in Eyebrows: A brow pencil was used to define and extend brows to the outer corners of Fern's eyes, where they should naturally end.

2. Hide Gray Strands: To prevent hair from looking thin, Fern will use a root touch-up kit between color appointments.

3. Part Hair Differently: Her bangs used to stick up, but switching Fern's part to the other side allows them to now fall softly across her forehead.

66
Going dark made my hair look thicker!"
–Fern

- **Add depth with color.** Dye is another route to lush locks. "Highlights and lowlights add dimension, making hair look thicker," says Rhys. Coloring also temporarily plumps the cuticle, so strands appear slightly fuller.

- **Consider clip-in extensions or hairpieces.** If you're still craving volume, you can try hair extensions, which have become much more affordable and easier to use in recent years. (See: Everything You Need to Know About Temporary Hair Extensions, p. 36.)

To Hide Thinning Areas...

- **Keep roots colored.** When hair is going gray, it blends in with the scalp. "So your hair actually looks thinner than it is, particularly at the roots," says David Kingsley, PhD, an expert in hair and scalp issues. The simple fix: In between shampoos, use a root concealer or temporary root touch-up wand to hide grays around your part. **TRY: Avon Advanced Techniques Color Protection Grey Root Touch-Up** ($7; *7yearsyounger.com/shop*) or **Color Wow Root Cover-Up** ($34; *7yearsyounger.com/shop*).

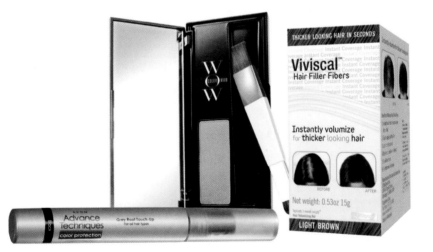

- **Try hair fibers.** Just like human hair, these fibers are made of protein and are an easy new option for concealing thinning areas on your scalp—especially a sparse part. Post-drying and -styling (you want to do this *last*), shake onto each area, then pat into your scalp. The electrostatically charged particles will bind to strands, creating a fuller, thicker look that lasts until you shampoo. (Tip: These products hold well and don't tend to flake off, but for insurance, lightly spray with a nonaerosol hairspray—this locks the fibers onto your hair.) **TRY: Viviscal Hair Filler Fibers** ($20, five shades; *7yearsyounger.com/shop*) or **Toppik Hair Building Fibers** ($26, nine shades; *7yearsyounger.com/shop*).

- **Don't rule out wigs.** First off, it's important to know that when hair is thinning from the scalp you should avoid clip-in extensions and hairpieces, which can tug at already weakened roots and damage hair follicles, leading to more hair loss. But the good news is, wigs are just a step up from extensions, and the styles have come a long way in recent years. Online sites like *wigs.com* offer a variety of options (a good synthetic-hair wig will run you somewhere between $100 to $250), as well as resources that can help you find the proper type and fit—depending on how often you plan to wear it and what kind of versatility you need. (For example, a wig made of human hair can be heat-styled and will last longer, but is more expensive.) Also, if you like to pull your hair back, you'll need a cap with lace at the crown—this provides a natural-looking hairline. But no matter what type of wig you buy, the number one trick for pulling it off, say experts, is this: Take it to your stylist and have it shaped to your face. (They may need to clean up a short style around your ears, for example.)

7 YEARS YOUNGER MAKEOVER
The Problem: Loss of Volume

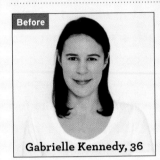
Before

Gabrielle Kennedy, 36

Is there a way to revamp your hairstyle but keep it low-maintenance? That's what Gabrielle, a freelance chef, wanted to know. After turning 35 and noticing her first few fine lines and gray strands, she was looking for a change. "My biggest problem area is my fine hair," she said. "It keeps getting thinner—I'd love to find the right cut that flatters my face, works with my texture and keeps me looking and feeling youthful."

THE FIX:

- **The Lob:** A mid-neck cut that's longer in the front and shorter in the back helps limp hair look thicker from all angles, says Taylor Fennema, a hairstylist at Oscar Blandi Salon. Tip: Ask for long layers, which gives hair bounce. (See: Get Layers, p. 52.)

- **Add Highlights:** Gabrielle said her go-to beauty product was bronzer, but colorist Kyle White at the Oscar Blandi Salon gave her a better way to brighten her complexion. He turned Gabrielle's hair to a lighter, medium brown hue with caramel highlights. The two tones added dimension, making her hair look fuller. (See: Pick the Perfect Shade, p. 43.)

FINISHING TOUCHES

1. Give Roots a Boost: To promote lift, Taylor applied a volumizing spray to Gabrielle's hairline and massaged it in.

2. Try Dry Shampoo: Between washes, Gabrielle will spray dry shampoo on roots and comb through to zap oil that weighs down her hair.

3. Apply Mascara: Black volumizing mascara helps draw attention to her eyes and open them up so she doesn't look tired.

*Layers gave
my thin hair
bounce."*
–Gabrielle

Everything You Need to Know About Temporary Hair Extensions

If you can't shell out for salon extensions that you wear full time (one row of weaving costs about $100, lasting six weeks), clip-in pieces are affordable and easy, and almost any brand will work, says Tina McIntosh, a hair extension and replacement artist at Shear Art Salon in Tampa, Florida.

1. Know your options. Extensions can be made of either human or synthetic hair. Synthetic hair is less expensive, usually can't be styled with heat, and needs to be replaced after two to three months of everyday wear. Human hair, on the other hand, costs up to three times as much, but it also lasts longer with everyday wear (six months to a year) and can be styled normally.

2. Shop smart. Match the hue to the very ends of your hair, and be sure the diameter of the hair strands is close to your own too. (If you're buying online, call and ask if the hair is thin or coarse). And if you choose human hair, look for the word Remy or virgin, which means it has been minimally processed.

3. Take it to your stylist. To really make your extensions work with your own style, take them to your next hair appointment, and ask your stylist to clip them in after she finishes cutting your hair. That way, she can shape them so they blend seamlessly with your haircut. It might cost extra, so call first to negotiate a price.

4. Clip it in correctly. Take your fingertips and divide out a section of hair from your eyes to the back of your head. Tie that section on top of your head, then tease the hair just below it to create traction; next, secure the clip on top (most simply snap on to hair). Drop hair down and gently comb to blend. Tip: Move the clip a quarter of an inch every time to prevent pulling in one place.

5. Keep it looking healthy. Each brand may sell its own line of cleansing products, but you can use what you already have, says McIntosh. Wash synthetic hair with a gentle laundry soap, and for human hair, put a quarter-size drop of shampoo in a large bowl filled with warm water. Gently dip to cleanse, then place it in a bowl of clean water to rinse. Repeat with conditioner. Both types can be hung on a pants hanger to dry. (That's also when you'll blow out or curl human-hair extensions—styling while clipped in can pull at roots and damage your scalp.)

FIX IT SO IT LASTS

Treat the Cause

First, the bad news: Once you start to experience genetic hair loss (also known as *androgenic alopecia*), there's not much you can do to grow back hair that's already gone, says Dr. Bank. Fortunately, hair loss caused by other factors—like stress, poor diet, medications, health problems and breakage—is usually completely reversible. How can you tell the difference?

- **Genetic hair loss:** This is usually a very slow, gradual process, and often there's a family history. "It's not common that you're going to see shedding," says Dr. Bank. "It's just that you look in the mirror and see more scalp staring back at you than before."

- **Systemic hair loss:** With all other types of hair loss, you'll notice a more abrupt thinning, with a greater number of strands collecting on your pillow, in your brush and in the drain after showering. It usually starts showing up about four to six months after the growth cycle is disrupted by something like extreme stress, illness or the start of a new medication.

TRY: Your Best Hair Extensions

- **Luxy Hair** is a budget-friendly source for shiny clip-in pieces made from Remy Human Hair ($129.95 and up for fine hair, 11 shades; *luxyhair.com*).

- **Hairdo by HairUWear** makes everything from bangs to full length clip-in extensions from polyester fibers ($29 and up; *hairuwear.com*).

- **Ultratress** is a line of 100 percent Remy Human Hair extensions, available at salons nationwide (prices vary; go to *ultratress.com* to find a participating stylist).

QUICK TIP

Prevent breakage.
Hair also loses elasticity with age, so you experience more of the brittleness and breakage that leads to thinner ends. (To keep hair soft, supple and safe from harsh styling treatments, See: Mini-Makeover #1, p. 13.)

The bottom line? "Either way, see a doctor right away who can help you figure out the cause," says Dr. Bank. For those with genetic hair loss, you might be able to start an over-the-counter topical treatment (like Minoxidil) that prevents further loss and wakes up dormant hair follicles. And with systemic hair loss, you can "fix the cause, which reboots the system and gets hair growing again," he adds. This may be as simple as tweaking your diet (See: Bonus Food Fix, *below*) or switching medications. You can also try an exfoliating treatment with salicylic acid, which might help unblock hair follicles, stimulate the scalp and promote hair growth. **TRY: Aveda Scalp Remedy Dandruff Solution** ($30; *7yearsyounger.com/shop*).

BONUS FOOD FIX
Eat for Thicker, Stronger Hair

Is your diet primed for healthy hair growth? Here's Dr. Kingsley's best advice:

1. Always add protein. Your body can't make hair without it, so be sure every single meal has fish, chicken, meat, tofu, eggs, chickpeas or beans. Bonus: These foods also pack a good mix of iron and B vitamins, which are essential for healthy hair too.

2. Don't skip meals. If energy isn't being delivered to your hair on a regular basis, the growth cycle gets disrupted, says Dr. Kingsley. That's why you need to eat every few hours, even if it's just a snack.

3. Take a multivitamin. One specially formulated for healthy hair growth will provide extra insurance that you're hitting all of the nutrients you need, like biotin and vitamin D (scientists are just now learning it's crucial for hair growth).

MINI-MAKEOVER #6
Go Gray the Right Way

Graying changes the health and texture of your hair, since pigment serves as a protective layer, making gray hair susceptible to damage. "It is instantly aging when gray hair looks frayed," says Cutler. But with the right cut and proper care routine, gray hair can look pretty and chic.

 Smooth the Transition

It's important to keep coloring until those silvery strands make up about 70 percent of your hair. Why? It's the salt-and-pepper stages that make hair look dull and old. When you're ready, here's how to do it.

- **Camouflage roots.** To avoid a contrast between graying roots and dyed hair, add highlights and lowlights (no more than two shades darker, within your natural color family), which will blend gray. Or cover up roots with a temporary concealer, which lasts until you shampoo. **TRY: Avon Advanced Techniques Color Protection Grey Root Touch-Up** ($7; *7yearsyounger.com/shop*).

- **Get a clever cut.** Experts agree that gray hair looks best above the shoulders, so try a chic bob with soft layers or a short pixie with a little volume on top. Not only will it speed up the process of growing in your gray, but it also sends the message that you're not letting yourself go. "You want to make a statement: 'This is my new look—I'm embracing my gray!'" says Hazan.

- **Tame your new texture.** Coloring hair smooths out the cuticle, so you'll need to add a little more polish to gray hair once you've stopped dying it all over. Use a shine-enhancer or smoothing product daily. (See: Your Best Frizz-Fighters, p. 22.)

7YEARS YOUNGER MAKEOVER
The Problem: Overgrown Grays

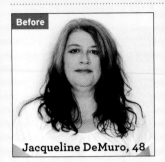
Before

Jacqueline DeMuro, 48

When Jacqueline signed up for the 7 Years Younger program, she had been growing out her gray for six months. "Dyeing every four weeks was drying out my hair, so I stopped," said the busy waitress and mom. "My hair was feeling better, but looked messy." Every time she considered going to the salon, though, she was afraid she'd be pressured to color again. The team at the Oscar Blandi Salon made her gray look stylish, not neglected.

THE FIX:

- **A Shoulder-Skimming Cut:** Jacqueline had old brown dye on the bottom half of her hair, so Taylor Fennema of the Oscar Blandi Salon cut off length to speed the transition. She also added side-swept bangs and longer layers to reduce the bulk in her hair. (See: Find Your Best Anti-Aging Cut, p. 52.)

- **A Better Blend:** Colorist Kyle White at the Oscar Blandi Salon added more gray to the white strands she already had coming in to blend the shades and make it look more natural as it grows in. (See: Go Gray the Right Way, p. 39.)

FINISHING TOUCHES

1. Wear a Bold Lip: Jacqueline traded in her nude and brown lipsticks for a shiny berry gloss, which instantly livened up her complexion.

2. Whiten Teeth: A professional whitening treatment helps remove stains that added years to her face.

3. Deep Condition Hair: Gray hair can lack luster. The experts recommend Jacqueline use a weekly hydrating hair mask to pep up her hair.

66

I'm glad I stayed gray—I love it!"

–Jacqueline

Keep It Shiny and Healthy

To look its best, gray, silver or white hair needs a boost. "Keep it up, just like a color or dye job," says Hazan. Here's how:

- **So color stays vibrant:** Because gray hair lacks melanin, it can pick up pigments from the environment (smoke in the air or minerals in the water), products (chemical relaxers are a big culprit) or the oils on your scalp. The result: Your hair looks dull or even turns a little yellow. To keep color pure and prevent tarnishing, make sure styling products are white or clear, and use a shampoo and conditioner specially formulated for gray hair once or twice a week. Since most have blue tones to balance out the yellow, everyday use could give you a violet tinge. **TRY: Klorane Shampoo with Centaury** ($15; 7yearsyounger.com/shop) or **Aveda Blue Malva Shampoo** ($31.50 for 1 liter; at salons).

- **To make it soft:** Gray hair tends to be drier and coarser, so when you're not using your blue-tinged products, switch to hydrating shampoo and conditioner. **TRY: Pantene Age Defy Shampoo and Conditioner** (each $8.99; at drugstores). Then, for extra smoothness, use a deep-conditioner once every two weeks, says Hazan. **TRY: Suave Professionals Moroccan Infusion Deep Conditioning Shine Mask** ($3; 7yearsyounger.com/shop).

- **To give it shine:** Gray hair does not reflect light on its own, so you need to add sheen. At your next trim, ask your stylist for a clear glaze (it generally costs $20 to $50, depending on the salon), or use an at-home shine gloss three times a week. Just apply the product after shampooing and conditioning, leave it in for 3 minutes, and rinse. **TRY: Rita Hazan Ultimate Shine Color Gloss in Clear** ($15; 7yearsyounger.com/shop).

MINI-MAKEOVER #7
Re-Do Your Hue

Your dye job might be aging you. "A woman's complexion becomes more translucent over time, so what looked great at 25 may not at 50," says celebrity stylist Nick Arrojo, owner of Arrojo Studio in New York City. The key is shifting to a softer, warmer shade with a little bit of depth.

 Pick the Perfect Shade

Subtle tweaks to your hair color can make a huge difference.

- **Go warmer.** Shift to a shade within the same color family you normally use that has gold or red in it to brighten your complexion. "Ashy tones tend to be matte, which is aging," says Hazan. Blondes can go for a honey or golden blond, while brunettes can try golden browns, chestnuts or auburns.

- **Make it multidimensional.** Dark, monotone hues create a harsh contrast with paling skin. Give hair depth and softness with multiple tones. If you're getting your hair colored at the salon, ask for a few subtle highlights around your face and part—these will also help to blend gray roots as they grow in. For at-home dying, choose a product that provides "multidimensional color" or "highlights and lowlights" in one step. **TRY: Clairol Nice 'N Easy with Color-Blend Technology** ($7.99, 44 shades; at drugstores).

- **Finish it off with a glaze.** Ask your stylist to apply a gloss or glaze, which gives it a silky sheen (most are free with color). "Have your stylist put you under the heat with it," says Rhys. "The heat opens up that cuticle layer and locks the color in, which gives you lasting shine for at least four weeks."

Keep Color Fresh and Vibrant

Keep a rich shade from fading quickly and losing its shine between dyes with these tips to make color last longer:

1 **Switch to color-protecting products.** Colorists agree that using shampoo and conditioner specially formulated for color-treated hair is nonnegotiable—they're less stripping than their standard counterparts. Don't wash every day, since frequent shampooing strips color too. **TRY: Suave Professionals Moroccan Infusion Color Care** ($4.59 each; *7yearsyounger.com/shop*) or **Color Wow Color Security Shampoo** ($22; *ulta.com*).

2 **Use a dry shampoo.** Formulated to absorb oil and bring back volume, it keeps hair fresh on days you don't wash it. **TRY: Garnier Fructis Volume Extend Instant Bodifier Dry Shampoo** ($6; *7yearsyounger.com/shop*).

3 **Add a glaze to your routine.** Chemically altering your hair color can lead to dryness, since the cuticle— it's what protects your hair—lifts during the process. A gloss that deposits pigment to boost color (or a clear one that simply seals the cuticle) will give you instant shine with minimal effort. Use it after you shampoo and condition, no more than three times a week. **TRY: John Frieda Luminous Glazes in Clear Shine Gloss or Brilliant Brunette**

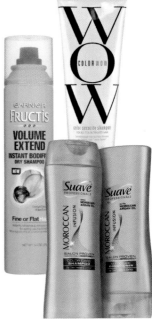

($7.99 each; *7yearsyounger.com/shop*) or **Rita Hazan Ultimate Shine Color Gloss in Clear** ($15; *7yearsyounger.com/shop*).

4 **Keep hair hydrated.** "Colored hair is dehydrated, because the process removes your natural oils," says Hazan. "So you have to put that moisture back." Most hair types only need a deep-conditioning treatment once a week to keep hair looking healthy, but if your hair is relaxed with chemicals or curly (curly hair is typically drier to begin with), you should consider increasing that to two or three times a week. Bonus: Moisturized hair will hold color longer too. **TRY: AGEbeautiful Intense Strengthening Treatment** ($8; *7yearsyounger.com/shop*).

5 **Protect locks from the sun.** Combat the sun's fading effects with a UV spray, which you can spray on damp or dry hair before you go outside. **TRY: L'Oréal Paris Advanced Haircare Color Vibrancy Dual Protect Spray** ($7; at CVS stores).

Keep Gray Covered

1. Reapply color every four to six weeks. For at-home color, you don't need to dye your whole head. Just divide your hair into sections and add color to the regrowth areas along the roots using a cotton swab.

2. Use a root touch-up kit in between. If pesky grays poke through early, this can buy a little extra time between colorings. **TRY: No Gray Quick Fix** ($5.99; 3 shades; *7yearsyounger.com/shop*) or **Color Wow Root Cover-Up** ($34; *7yearsyounger.com/shop*).

3. Get the right cut. Ask your stylist for soft, side-swept front layers or a long bang that you can brush to the side. These help cover the grays that appear along the hairline, says New York City hairstylist Patrick Melville. And the face-framing effect is an instant youth boost, no matter your age.

Get Amazing Color at Home

Going more than three shades lighter or darker than your natural base should always be done in a salon. But for enhancing your natural color, you can get salon-quality results with these pro pointers.

STEP ONE: Pick the right product.

You'll want to hide gray by coloring your hair with a product that is ammonia-free. This means it doesn't contain harsh chemicals, says celebrity hairstylist Andre Walker.

- **Permanent dyes** lift color from hair, then lighten or darken it one to two shades. They provide great gray coverage, but require upkeep to deal with root regrowth. **TRY: Garnier Olia Oil Powered Permanent Color** ($7.99; *7yearsyounger.com/shop*).

- **Demi-permanent** will fade after about 25 shampoos, so roots are less of an issue. **TRY: Clairol Natural Instincts** ($5, 32 shades; *7yearsyounger.com/shop*)

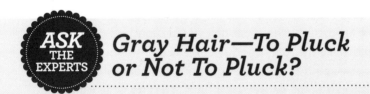

ASK THE EXPERTS — *Gray Hair—To Pluck or Not To Pluck?*

Yanking out a gray hair once in a while is probably fine, says Dr. Kingsley. (There's zero truth to the old adage that two will grow back in its place.) Still, don't make it a habit. "The more you pluck, the greater the chance that you damage those hair follicles," he adds, "and those hairs won't grow back at all." The bottom line: If thinning becomes a concern, you may need those hairs–gray or not!

- **Semipermanent** is color-depositing only (you can't make hair lighter) and will wash out after four to eight shampoos. **TRY: L'Oréal Paris Healthy Look Crème Gloss** ($9; *drugstore.com*).

TIP: Always pick up two kits. If your hair is very thick or long, one box may not be enough. (If you don't use the second one, you should be able to return it to the store, or save it for the next time you color.)

STEP TWO: Color with care.

These five steps will keep hair healthy and make color last.

1 **Skip the shampoo.** Don't wash your hair for 24 hours before coloring or you'll remove the oils that protect your scalp from the chemicals. (And rinse out the dye with water only—shampoo can strip color.)

2 **Be sure to condition.** Use a deep-conditioning mask the day before you dye. It will help ward off any damage, and color looks more vibrant and deposits more evenly on moisturized hair.

3 **Read the directions.** Many women ignore them or just go by the pictures. Pay close attention to the processing time. Leaving dye on for even a few minutes too long can give very different results.

4 **Do a strand test.** It's the only way to see how the color will really develop on your hair. Snip a small section at the nape of your neck (where hair tends to be darkest) and apply the product as directed.

5 **Apply color evenly.** Divide your hair into four or five manageable sections using clips or elastics. Starting with the lower sections, unclip, apply the product generously from roots to ends, then move up to the next section.

MINI-MAKEOVER #8
Update Your Hairstyle

It's so easy to stick to your same old cut, especially if you feel like you've got the styling routine down. But this comfort zone can make you appear dated. "If you have the same 'do you had 10 years ago, it's time for a new look," says Arrojo. Don't worry—you don't have to chop it all off. Even tiny tweaks, like switching up your blow-dry routine, will breathe life into your appearance.

FIX IT FAST **Try a Youth-Boosting Style**
It's OK if you're still leery of making a drastic change. There are simple ways you can switch your hairstyle almost instantly. Try one of these ideas:

1 **Change your part.** It seems so simple, but it works, especially if you have been parting your hair in the middle. (Middle parts can look severe and aging, say pros.) The key: Push hair opposite of the direction it grows in to add volume, says Cutler. "You get a natural swoop on top of the head, which lifts the eye." Plus, if you've been parting your hair in one place for years, that part may look thinner than it would elsewhere, thanks to repeated styling and combing at those roots, says Dr. Fusco.

2 **Try a gentle ponytail.** If your hair is mid-length or longer, wearing it off your face once in a while isn't just a nice, unexpected change—it can also give you a more chiseled appearance, if you keep it soft and give it a little lift at the roots. To get the perfect age-appropriate pony:

- First, add volume that will draw the eye up by softly teasing back-to-back, 2-inch wide sections of hair at the crown. Just lift hair straight up toward the ceiling and brush it down to the root with a paddle brush (two easy strokes on each section should do it).

- Then, gently pull hair back into a ponytail that's in line with the top of your ears. "Any higher, and it will seem like you're trying to look 16," says Rhys. Use your hand to smooth out the top, and secure it with a no-damage hair elastic to prevent breakage.

- To finish, rub a drop of a lightweight, moisturizing hair cream between your hands (shine serums are too heavy here) and apply it only to your ends. "This adds polish and hides split strands without weighing down the whole pony," Rhys adds.

3 **Blow longer hair back.** When hair is heavy and tucked in around the cheeks, it can draw attention to a sagging jawline. "Lifting the hair away from the face will bring out your eyes and accentuate your cheekbones—especially if you've got medium-length or long hair," says Cutler. The best time to do this is when you blow-dry: Apply a root booster to damp hair, then use your hand to lift the section of hair closest to the corner of your eyes and cheekbones off the scalp and up toward the ceiling. Then, blow up to the ends. "This points the roots in an antigravity direction, setting hair off the face," he adds.

4 **Give your bob swing.** "Nothing is more aging than over-styling!" says Rhys. (This is the danger with a bob—too many women curl it under and spray it, so that it's like a helmet.) If your hair grazes your chin or sits above your shoulders, making it move more can

7 YEARS YOUNGER MAKEOVER
The Problem: Shapeless Hair

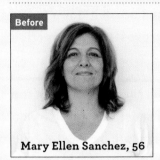

Before

Mary Ellen Sanchez, 56

Newly an empty-nester, Mary Ellen—a mom of three kids who works full-time as the chairperson of a local school district's special education program—decided it was time to make her outer appearance match the youthfulness she feels inside. "I want to look as young as I feel," she says. On her wish list: an updated cut and shiny hair, which has a fine texture and has thinned out considerably over the last two decades.

THE FIX:

- **A Youth-Boosting Haircut:** "She has amazing bone structure!" says stylist Nunzio Saviano. To make her length work for her, he gave her a chin-grazing cut with soft layers around the face, which acted as an instant facelift! (See: Find Your Best Anti-Aging Cut, p. 52.)

- **Complexion-Brightening Color:** Stephanie Brown, a colorist at the Nunzio Saviano salon, says Mary Ellen's hair matched her skin tone, which did nothing to brighten her face. So after applying a single-process color to hide grays, Brown added blond highlights. (See: Pick the Perfect Shade, p. 43.)

FINISHING TOUCHES

1. Apply a Heat Protective Spray: Mary Ellen's blow-dry style needs protection from the color-fading heat.

2. Line Eyes: Side-swept bangs softly brush against her eyes, drawing attention to them. Defining their shape with liner helps make them pop.

3. Try a Boar Bristle Brush: Instead of using a flat iron, Mary Ellen learned to smooth out hair with a round brush, which also minimizes heat damage.

The body in my hair took years off my face!"
—Mary Ellen

soften your facial features. Her best advice? Next time you blow-dry, trade your round brush for a paddle brush and use her "windshield wiper" method: Divide hair down the middle of the back of your head, and blow each section toward your face until it's 85 percent dry. Then, finish by blowing hair back in the opposite direction. "It's an all-in-one solution," says Rhys. "It removes wiriness and gives hair swing."

5 **Add separation to a short cut.** If you've got a cropped 'do or bob and typically finish it with a spray, experiment with whips or pomades, which add texture and lift, says Shorter. **TRY: Toni&Guy Hair Meet Wardrobe Creative Stick It Up Gum** ($15; at Target stores).

6 **Rethink tight, slicked-back or too-youthful styles.** Anything that keeps hair tight against the scalp—like an extremely sleek bun or flat twists—can appear harsh against aging skin. "You want softness as you age," says Garcia-Jackson.

Find Your Best Anti-Aging Cut

Is your haircut aging you? Certain cuts can accentuate the signs of aging, while others can counter the changes you're seeing on and around your face. Here are a few tweaks—some subtle, others a bit more bold—that stylists say you might want to consider:

1 **Get layers.** Every stylist we talked to agreed: Hair that's all one length is heavy and can make you look tired, but adding at least a few soft, face-framing layers gives your features lightness and lift. (This is especially important if you want to keep your hair length below your shoulders.) "Adding layers really opens everything up and brings out the eyes," says Cutler. What's more: Layers are an easy way to give volume a boost.

2 **Switch up the length.** Hair that's too long (even if it's thinning or doesn't have much body) can weigh down your face, while hair that hits at the chin might draw more attention to a sagging jawline. A cut that grazes the collarbone, though, is universally flattering. It works on all hair types and textures, plus it can draw attention away from an aging neck, says Rhys. Many stylists also say cropped cuts that are a little longer on top can look modern and youthful, but only when they're sleek. "Too many women think a short cut is a free pass to forgo styling, but when hair has no polish, it can look matronly," Rhys says.

3 **Embrace your texture.** If you want to let your kinky or curly hair be natural, go for it—transitioning will take time (See: Tips for Transitioning Relaxed Hair, p. 24), but eventually, that soft base of curls is an instant youth-booster, says Shorter. If you already have curls, cut hair shoulder-length or above with some layering, then add highlights to create dimension. "Too much length on any texture can tend to be too heavy, but on textured hair specifically, longer hair will grow out instead of down," says Shorter. "This can make the face and frame look larger."

4 **Soften sharp edges.** Severe cuts that create harsh lines can accentuate wrinkles, so if you have a bob—or are considering one— you want to make sure the ends are soft and loose. Tell your stylist

7 YEAR YOUNGER MAKEOVER
The Problem: Lifeless Hair

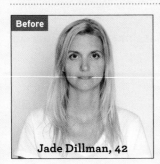
Before

Jade Dillman, 42

For Jade, a stay-at-home mom of five kids between the ages of 11 and 19, turning 40 hit harder than she expected. "I started noticing everything changing all at once," she says. Among her biggest concerns: limp, washed out hair and forehead wrinkles that frustrated her daily. "My hair's growing in gray, dry, and—while it's always been thin—it's now harder to style than ever," she explained. "I'm tired of my daily ponytail."

THE FIX:

- **Create Body and Bounce:** Fine hair appears fuller when it's above the shoulders, which is why Taylor Fennema, a stylist at the Oscar Blandi Salon, gave Jade a collarbone-grazing cut with long layers. "Shorter layers make thin hair look stringy, but these create movement and bounce," she says. (See: Get Layers, p. 52.)

- **Avoid Going Too Blond:** Colorist Kyle White at the Oscar Blandi Salon said Jade's hair color was washing her out. He made her base champagne blond and mixed in both one shade deeper and one shade lighter to warm up her look and create definition.

FINISHING TOUCHES

1. Update a Ponytail: Jade's new wispy fringed bangs help hide forehead lines and will add softness to her go-to ponytail style.

2. Define Features with Bronzer: To warm up Jade's fair complexion makeup artist Sue Pike applied a light dust of bronzer to cheeks, jawline and along her hairline.

3. Curl Eye Lashes: Instead of relying on mascara to do all the work, curling Jades's long lashes help to wake up her blue eyes.

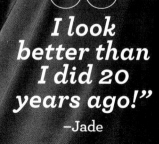

I look better than I did 20 years ago!"
–Jade

Slash costs on hair services. Three smart ways to cut your beauty budget at the salon:

1. Book with a junior stylist. If you're wary of taking advantage of cheap cuts at your local beauty school, this is a safer alternative. "Junior stylists and colorists charge much less, but work under the supervision of senior staff members," says Hazan.

2. Go on a slow day. "If your salon is open on Mondays—many aren't—it's probably slowest," says Hazan. "So it's likely you'll be given a discount, or even complimentary services." (Savings we found by asking around: 15 percent off a color treatment or blowout, and a $50 cut, color and style for first-time clients.)

3. Inquire about freebies. Even if your salon doesn't advertise them, ask anyway, says Barbara Fazio, owner of Cleveland's B. Fazio salon. "I do free brow shapings with cuts, and some stylists offer free bang trims."

you want it "point cut," which means they'll hold the scissors vertically, taking little notches out along the ends. "It releases the bulk of the line, making the bob more free and moveable," says Rhys. Same goes for cropped cuts: Ask for a softer shape that will work well finger-styled and tousled. "You want it to look wispy, not spiky," adds Shorter.

5 **Try bangs.** Bangs can camouflage forehead lines (the "Bangtox" effect), but not all types do it equally well. "A blunt bang that hangs straight across the forehead isn't for everyone. It can emphasize aging features," says celebrity hairstylist Sarah Potempa. "Opt for a side-swept fringe with layers that blend into the rest of your hair; it'll make your features look more youthful." Rhys adds that these bangs should still be a bit wispy, rather than one solid swoop. "You want to see a little skin peeking through," she says. "That way it doesn't *look* like you're trying to hide something—but you still are!"

The Quickie Guide to Amazing Hair

If you do nothing else, try one or all of these tips for younger-looking hair.

1. Check Your Products Your texture is changing, so your shampoo and conditioner probably should too! Get ones specific to your new hair type or consider an anti-aging line, which is formulated to tackle multiple aging-related issues.

2. Deep Condition The scalp's oil glands slow down as you age, but a weekly hair mask will infuse strands with extra moisture to keep them soft and manageable.

3. Lift the Roots It's natural for hair to get finer and thinner, but it can't always hold curl or volume at the ends. If locks look limp. blow-dry hair up at the roots first, or use rollers to boost body around your part.

4. Add Polish Frizzy, dull hair will tack on years. To smooth it out and give it luster, find a treatment (like a gloss or glaze) or a finishing product (like a shine-enhancer) you love.

5. Warm Up Your Color Reddish or golden-tinged hues give hair vibrancy and bring out skin's glow. And making that color multidimensional (meaning it has a few highlights or different tones) will look more natural and youthful too.

6. Style Safely Hair is finer and more brittle than it used to be, and breakage contributes to thinning. So be mindful of brushes that tug, and if you must style with curling irons or flat irons, use a low setting and a heat-protectant spray.

7. Get Bangs and/or Layers Cuts that are harsh or all one length weigh down your face, but these tiny tweaks add instant softness and lift. (And get a trim every six to eight weeks so thinning ends look polish, not frayed!)

Refresh Your Face **2**

How to even out skin tone, hide wrinkles, recapture that natural glow and give your face an instant lift—no surgery required.

66 **The face you have at 25 is the face God gave you, but the face you have after 50 is the face you earned."** — *Cindy Crawford*

A ging changes occur before we can see them," says Jeanette Graf, MD, dermatologist and author of *Stop Aging, Start Living.* "But they don't typically become apparent until our late 30s and 40s." The unavoidable mix of your genetics and the passage of time is simply the natural aging process. Your skin's production of collagen and elastin—the proteins responsible for its structure and elasticity—starts to slow, so "skin gets more lax, losing its shape," explains Elizabeth Tanzi, MD, a dermatologist in Washington, DC.

This isn't meant to be scary. Instead, it should give you a clear picture of what's happening beneath the surface, not only to demystify the aging process (remember, it's happening to everyone!) but also to help you eventually understand how and why these targeted treatments and tricks we're suggesting will work. In this chapter, you'll find skincare tips and makeup strategies for your overall complexion—how to create a fresh, rosy glow with makeup, soften forehead lines, shrink your pores, and more. Ready to take years off your face? Here we go!

MINI-MAKEOVER #1
Give Your Face a Lift

Does your face feel droopy? As women age, many may start to notice a shift in shape: Their cheeks lose some plumpness, the temples hollow out and the skin slides downward, eventually causing loose skin to gather around the jawline. So what's going on? "You intrinsically lose a teaspoon of volume from your face every year from the time you are 30," says Jeanine Downie, MD, director of Image Dermatology in Montclair, New Jersey. Pair this natural fat loss with external damage from sun and/or smoking, and your face now lacks some of its original elasticity. So it softens—and sinks.

 Define and Lift

The quick, right-now solution for sagging skin involves some simple contouring, a little added brightness, and carefully placed blush, which will "lift, lift, lift," says celebrity makeup artist Joanna Schlip. Here's how to accentuate your jawline and use products that catch light in all the right places. Your face will look shapelier—and your skin more radiant.

1 Start with your base of choice: a liquid foundation, BB cream or tinted moisturizer will even out your skin's tone and texture. (See: Find Your Best Base, p. 73.) "I like something with a little luminosity, because it softens any lines," says Schlip. Make sure you go all the way down to your neck (beneath your jawline), and behind your ears; this will "catch" all sagging skin to even out your canvas. **TRY: Physicians Formula Super BB All-in-1 Beauty Balm Cream** ($11; *7yearsyounger.com/shop*).

2 Once your foundation is dry, lightly brush a matte bronzer that's two shades darker than your skin tone in a "3" shape along one side of your face: Starting in the middle of your forehead, take it along the hairline; bring it down underneath the cheekbone; pull it out again; then brush it beneath the jawbone. (You want to see contour, but if the line is *too* defined, buff the edge by going over it with your brush, in a circular motion.) Repeat on the other side. This will give your face the illusion of a more defined structure, says Schlip, while adding depth. **TRY: Sephora Collection Bronzer** ($17; *sephora.com*)

3 Now, finish with a bright but soft blush in a shade like poppy, coral or pink. Smile first, then place blush only on the apple of your cheek, using fingers to rub it in—but not out. You want to keep the brightness concentrated there, for that lifting effect, explains Schlip. **TRY: Maybelline New York Dream Bouncy Blush** ($7.99; at drugstores).

BONUS BEAUTY FIX
Perfect the Bold Brow

A well-shaped and properly filled eyebrow will frame your face and also give sagging skin the appearance of an instant lift. (See: Create Face-Framing Brows, p. 114.)

BONUS HAIR FIX
Give Your Face an Instant Lift

Worried about saggy skin or jowls? These tips will help defy gravity.

- **Try an updo.** If your hair is longer, wearing it off your face can give you a more defined appearance. For shorter hair, using a root-lifting spray can achieve the same effect. (For specific tutorials, See: Try a Youth-Boosting Style, p. 48.)

- **Cut to flatter.** Hair that grazes the collarbone—with a few soft layers—will hide an aging neck and emphasize your bone structure. (For more haircut advice, See: Find Your Best Anti-Aging Cut, p. 52.)

Moisturize, Protect, Firm

Some extra moisture and diligent defense from UV rays—along with a few key firming and rejuvenating ingredients—can help lift and tighten skin. Here, your best laid plan:

STEP ONE: Protect.

Slather on a moisturizer with SPF every morning.

According to dermatologists, skin that's kept moist will appear smoother, younger and more supple, while SPF will slow down collagen and elastin loss, no matter how much damage you've already done. So buy sunscreen and use it—always. "Before you even think about spending money on fancy creams and treatments, you really have to be committed to keeping the sun off your face," says Dr. Tanzi. Products that repair damage are pointless if you don't prevent the same type of damage they're trying to correct. (See: Save Face!,p. 67.) Here, you might want to consider an extra-hydrating, anti-aging formula that includes retinol, which can firm

The Problem: Sagging Skin

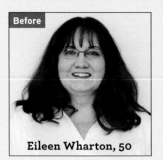

Before

Eileen Wharton, 50

Eileen, a single mom to three kids in their early 20s, also works three jobs. "I'm always putting myself last," she says. But her 50th birthday kickstarted her desire to fix the skin issues that have been troubling her. Eileen was frustrated by the changes happening to her face—age spots, droopy jowls, disappearing eyebrows and little lines around her mouth. "I want to start the second half of my life as a new woman," she says.

THE FIX:

- **The Right Cut:** Eileen was sensitive to the sagging skin around her jawline, and her hair was too long and overgrown, and "the weight of her thick strands was dragging her features down," says hairstylist Nunzio Saviano, of Nunzio Saviano Salon. He gave Eileen a shoulder-skimming cut with lots of layers, which lifted her face. (See: Give Your Face an Instant Lift, p. 63.)

- **Cheeks That Pop:** Makeup artist Sue Pike applied blush on the apples of Eileen's cheeks, then brushed bronzer underneath her cheekbones, blending it up with her fingers. This contouring trick subtracted years. (See: Define and Lift, p. 61.)

FINISHING TOUCHES

1. Face-framing Highlights: Eileen's caramel streaks blend perfectly with her rich chocolate base to brighten up her complexion.

2. Use Eyebrow Powder: In the past, she'd just pencil in her thinning brows, but adding powder over the top will make them look natural, not severe.

3. Apply Shine Spray: Eileen's bouncy, healthy locks got a radiance boost. A few spritzes also helped tame flyaways.

66
I look amazing and feel great!"
−Eileen

skin—but only if you aren't using it elsewhere in your regimen. (See: Ask the Experts: What's Retinol?, p. 70.) **TRY: Neutrogena Rapid Wrinkle Repair Moisturizer SPF 30** ($18.69; *7years younger.com/shop*). Good Housekeeping Research Institute testers say it improved skin tone, softened fine lines *and* firmed skin, while also dispensing a good dose of hydration.

STEP TWO: REJUVENATE

Zero in on firming and rejuvenating ingredients. Some docs say that the only thing that will help firm sagging skin are anti-aging treatments that stimulate collagen production, which could help restore part of your skin's natural suppleness and structure. So look for creams or serums that contain retinoids (like retinol), peptides (milder but less effective than retinoids) or growth factors (highly effective but pricey). You can use a lighter product that you apply in the morning, like the SPF day cream mentioned above or an anti-aging serum that you apply before your moisturizer. **TRY: Olay Regenerist Micro-Sculpting Serum** ($16.99; *7yearsyounger.com/shop*). At the very least, though, you'll want to dedicate yourself to a nighttime treatment containing one or more of these collagen-building ingredients. (Here's why: Your skin repairs itself while you sleep, which might make aging-fighters extra effective.)

Save Face! Your Guide to SPF

Think you don't need it every day? "The *aha* moment for many of my patients is when I tell them to take a look at the skin on their face, versus the skin on their bum," adds Dr. Tanzi. "That gives you a good idea of the damage the sun can do." But the sea of SPF-laced face products out there can make your head spin. Here's how to choose the right one for the right situation—and use it correctly.

1. Pick your protection. Always choose a sunscreen that's SPF 30 to 50—look for broad spectrum, which means it protects from both UVA and UVB rays.

2. Pick your product. You can never go wrong with a plain sunscreen, but certain multitasking creams and powders can ease your routine. To make sure you're covered:

- **If you're going to be outside...**sunscreen-only products are your best bet. These potent potions provide your strongest protection—best for beach days, poolside lounging, outdoor exercise and whenever you'll be soaking up the sun's sneaky rays for more than a few minutes. A facial formula will feel lighter, but always choose one that's labeled water-resistant or very water-resistant. That way, it works while sweating or swimming too.

- **If you'll only see the sun briefly...**your SPF-infused foundation, BB cream or moisturizer (as long as its SPF 30 or above) should do the job. This is for days spent mostly inside, with a few quick errands. "The SPF in makeup gets diluted," says Dr. Tanzi. (The main reason: You usually don't apply it as thickly as you would a lotion that seeps into your skin.)

- **If you need to touch it up...**and are already wearing makeup, try a powder with sunscreen. "Many women I talk to hate to reapply because they don't want to get greasy," says Dr. Tanzi. "But you can apply these powders right over your makeup."

3. Put it on. For liquids or creams, apply about a tablespoon, to your face, neck and chest each morning. (See: Erase Years from Your Neck and Chest, p. 154.) Reapply every 2 hours, or after you take a dip in the water.

7 YEARS YOUNGER MAKEOVER
The Problem: Dull Complexion

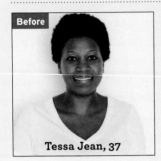

Before

Tessa Jean, 37

Shortly after being one of the first testers of the *7 Years Younger Anti-Aging Plan* a little over two years ago, Tessa, then 35, learned she was pregnant. She credits 7 Years Younger with helping her bounce back quickly after giving birth. The good sleep habits saved her, she explains. Still, the hospital administrator—who has her skincare regimen down pat from last time around—wanted to refresh her makeup to keep her look current.

THE FIX:

- **A Filled-in Brow:** The Laura Geller Makeup team colored in her brows, using tiny strokes in the direction of hair growth—for a longer, thicker line that frames her face and balances her big, beautiful brown eyes. (See: Create a Face-Framing Brow, p. 114.)

- **Wear a Bold Lipcolor:** After lining Tessa's lips to give them definition, Geller's team applied a bright pink gloss to help bring out the whiteness of Tessa's teeth, making her beautiful smile a focal point. (See: Brighten Your Lips, p. 142.) A little blush concentrated on the apples of her cheeks also helped to wake up her face.

FINISHING TOUCHES

1. **Apply Translucent Powder:** A light dusting across Tessa's skin helped minimize shininess without ruining her makeup.
2. **Put on Sparkling Eyeshadow:** To help liven up eyes, shimmery silver shadow was applied from the lash line to the crease of Tessa's lids.
3. **Use a Facial Spray:** Tessa can spritz on a facial spray to freshen up skin and makeup throughout her busy day.

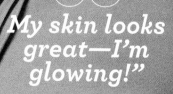

My skin looks great—I'm glowing!"

–Tessa

What's Retinol?

Ah, yes. This star anti-aging ingredient—a vitamin A derivative—is everywhere these days, and with good reason. It's a proven wrinkle fighter, and it (and other retinoids) will stimulate the production of collagen and decrease its breakdown, helping to minimize and prevent fine lines. Retinol also speeds up cell turnover, so it's effective for fading dark spots too. But there are a few other things you should know before you use it:

- **Start with drugstore products.** Prescription-strength retinoid acid is stronger and can give you better results, but it can also be more irritating, so it's usually best to start with retinol. Not only will your skin have a chance to acclimate to the ingredient, but it's also much less expensive—so you'll spend less money figuring out if you can tolerate the ingredient. (Many women can't—it's strong, especially on sensitive skin—and that's OK. Other anti-aging ingredients, like peptides and vitamin C, also have wrinkle-fighting benefits.)

- **Be careful in the sun.** Retinol makes you more susceptible to burning and irritation from sunlight. That goes for the whole time you're using a retinol, and for several weeks after you stop—whether you put it on in the morning or at night. This is because speedier cell turnover pushes newer, more delicate skin to the surface. Sunscreen is (as always) a must.

- **It works best at night.** The theory is that your skin is repairing itself then, so any anti-aging products you apply will be more effective. And sunlight has been thought to degrade retinol, decreasing its effectiveness. That doesn't mean you can't use it during the day, but when you start out, apply your retinol-infused product only at night. That way, if you experience dryness, stinging or redness as your skin adjusts, you'll sleep right through it. You can always add a day product once you are sure you don't see any of these side effects.

MINI-MAKEOVER #2
Restore Your Natural Glow

It's not uncommon for your face to lose a little of its luster as you get older, and part of that is sun damage, says Dr. Downie. But what's also at work here is a lack of moisture (skin produces less oil as we get older) and a slower rate of cell turnover. "When you're in your 20s, the normal life cycle of your skin is 28 days," says Ellen Marmur, MD, a dermatologist in New York City. "That gets longer in your 30s and 40s—which means you don't shed that top layer of dead skin naturally." The result: Less allover glow.

 Create a Rosy Radiance

According to makeup artist Laura Geller, there are a few common misconceptions and mistakes that might be holding you back from getting that dewy, youthful look. "Most women don't know how to bring back the brightness to their skin and recapture that vitality," she says. "They think it's all about foundation or bronzer, but you really need to start with texture—meaning primers with some shimmer or glow."

Geller also sees women struggle with choosing and applying the proper blush, which—according to her—is the secret to a rosy, natural-looking radiance. "When you smile and you have that color in the apple of the cheek, you get that pinched-cheek look that everybody's trying to retain from their youth," she says. "It's the easiest, quickest way to restore a beautiful, soft glow." To get it right, follow this simple tutorial:

1 **Use your face moisturizer first,** allowing cream to sink in for at least 30 seconds. This is crucial: Well-hydrated skin will appear plumper, with a bit of a dewy sheen.

2 Then, apply a thin layer of illuminating under-makeup primer all over: "These products have ingredients that reflect light, which will blur imperfections and give your skin instant vitality." **TRY: Hard Candy Sheer Envy Illuminating Primer** ($8; at Walmart stores).

3 Next step: Apply a cream foundation with a light texture, which will allow luminosity to shine through. Geller says many BB creams and CC creams (See: Find Your Best Base, p. 73) work well here—their extra moisture makes them a little lighter than typical foundation formulas. **TRY: L'Oréal Paris Visible Lift CC Cream** ($10.70; *7yearsyounger.com/shop*).

ASK THE EXPERTS

But What About Bronzer?

Some makeup artists *do* say that bronzer can give you that healthy, natural glow—and it's an especially good age-shaving option in the summer months, when you want to create the effect of a tan. The problem: If you're trying to correct dullness, you can overdo it with bronzer. But if you want to give bronzer a try to restore radiance, you need a non-shimmery one that's close to your skin tone. First brush it around the perimeter of your face: from below each ear to your jaw, then from temple to temple along the hairline. "I know it sounds nuts to focus on the outside of your face, but it's key to making the color look real," says celebrity makeup artist Mally Roncal. After that, gently dust the bronzer (tap off any excess color—you want a really light hand here!) on your cheekbones, nose, and chin, before finishing with a pop of pink blush on the apples of your cheeks.

4 Now take a brush and dip it into your powder blush. Pinks are universally flattering for all skin tones, says Geller—whether it's a shade of rose, cranberry or berry. Tap off the excess so you start with less, not more. (You can always go back and apply again, if need be!) Smile, then swirl it only on the apple of your cheek.

Find Your Best Base

The first rule of foundation: Swap out powder for a liquid or cream (they're more forgiving on aging skin). Here's what you need to know about your options:

Foundation: Traditional liquid or cream foundations vary greatly, but they'll give you your fullest coverage, even the sheer formulas. The makeup artists we talked to generally suggested you choose one with a little luminosity (look for words like luminous, illuminating or brightening) to boost dull, dry skin and soften lines. But if visible pores are your issue, go for one marked oil-free.

BB creams: Most "beauty balms" combine moisturizer, foundation, sunscreen and skincare (ingredients and benefits differ by brand) all in one. They're great for daytime wear—when you want something lighter than foundation but heavier than a tinted moisturizer—with one caveat: Their shade range is often limited.

CC Creams: Like BB creams, most CC ("color-correcting") creams deliver moisturizers, foundation and SPF in a limited number of shades, but there are two subtle differences: Their skincare ingredients are usually sunspot-fading vitamins, and their coverage is typically lighter and more natural than BB creams. (Textures and weight of each, however, differ by brand—so be sure to test first.)

Tinted moisturizer: The name explains it all: It'll hydrate skin and give you some color that evens out your complexion. This is the sheerest of the bunch, for light coverage. If it doesn't have SPF 30, make sure you apply sunscreen beforehand.

QUICK TIP

Try this pick-me-up. According to a study, women look oldest at 3:30 P.M. That's when stress levels peak and energy plummets, leaving skin dry, ruddy and dull. So every afternoon, pat lotion on your cheeks and under your eyes. Bonus points for soothing ingredients like chamomile and anti-inflammatories, like rosa gallica. **TRY: Kiehl's Skin Rescuer Stress-Minimizing Hydrator ($40; kiehls.com).**

FIX IT SO IT LASTS

Restore That Natural Glow

To get your glow back, always keep your face well-moisturized day and night, and be sure to slather on SPF every morning and throughout the day—that's almost a given (See: Save Face!, p. 67). But because you can't count on your skin to shed its dullness on its own, you need to help the process along with some gentle exfoliation, says Dr. Tanzi. (Exfoliation removes dead cells on the skin's surface, either by physically sloughing them off with a scrub or brush or by applying a product containing a chemical ingredient that loosens them until they fall off.) "A lot of the best products that exfoliate use glycolic acid," she says. "You can use those either in a serum form—or in a cream at night." If you have normal to oily sky, you can probably exfoliate every day, but sensitive skin types should only do it once or twice a week—and use products specially formulated to prevent irritation (look for exfoliators that say they're for sensitive skin or rosacea). "The cumulative effect is almost like having a light chemical peel in the office," says Dr. Tanzi. "You keep

TRY: DIY Dullness Fighter

Try this recipe, courtesy of celebrity facialist Joanna Vargas:
Yogurt-Grapefruit Mask Mix ½ cup plain yogurt; ½ cup corn meal; ¼ cup grapefruit juice. Cool in fridge to thicken, scrub onto face for two minutes, and rinse. **Cost per recipe: 47¢**

seeing the skin's healthy, fresh glow." For an everyday scrub, **TRY: Suki Exfoliate Foaming Cleanser** ($32.95; *sukiskincare.com*). For sensitive skin, **TRY: Simple Smoothing Facial Scrub** ($6; *7yearsyounger.com/shop*).

MINI-MAKEOVER #3
Smooth Out Forehead Lines

Here's why the furrows that form across your forehead and those vertical wrinkles between your brows are so frustrating: They often send a mistaken message to the world ("I'm angry!" "I'm grumpy!") that doesn't quite match up with how you really feel inside. But they are, indeed, a result of years and years of frowning or squinting. "You're not as young as you used to be, your collagen is not as thick, and your sun damage is catching up

---

BONUS FASHION FIX
Bring out your glow

Dull day? To lift your complexion and brighten your face, try these tips from *Woman's Day* Style Editor, Donna Duarte-Ladd:

- **Pull on a pink top.** It'll highlight the rosy tones in your skin and play up the effects of blush.

- **Wear gemstone jewelry.** Choose medium-length drop earrings and necklaces with embellishments. They'll attract light, which reflects off your skin, brightening your complexion.

- **Try a cheery scarf.** Wrapping a vivid shade like turquoise or coral around your neck can instantly perk you up and bring out the color in your eyes and cheeks.

to you," says Dr. Downie. "So all of a sudden you're 40 or 50 and you're frowning, and—boom! You're seeing these lines and wrinkles that you've never had before." What's more: Loss of moisture as you get older (the skin isn't producing as much oil as it used to) can make them appear even deeper.

Prime and Illuminate

If it's forehead lines you're worried about, then a few makeup tricks can make deep creases seem to vanish, says Schlip:

1 Start with a silicone-based primer, "which acts like spackle to fill in the creases," she says. First, gently rub a pea-size drop between your index finger and thumb, to warm it up. Then, apply it with your fingers, pushing it into the wrinkles and blending it in. **TRY: L'Oréal Paris RevitaLift Miracle Blur Instant Skin Smoother and Finishing Cream** ($14.43; *7yearsyounger.com/shop*) or **Laura Geller Beauty Spackle Under Make-Up Primer** ($27.95; *7yearsyounger.com/shop*).

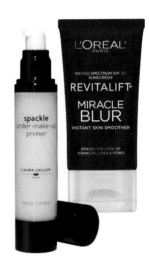

2 Top it with a dab of liquid foundation, then trace the tip of a skin-toned eye pencil inside the crevice of the wrinkle. "This makes the line appear more shallow," she says. **TRY: Baby Eyes Enhancer by Paula Dorf Cosmetics** ($20; *pauladorf.com*).

3 Pat the area with loose powder, then play up your lips. "A bold lipstick will take the focus away from your forehead," she says.

HABIT REHAB
Let Your Face Relax

Guess what? The less you frown or squint, the fainter forehead lines will be. Try these expert tips and see for yourself.

1. Raise your electronics to eye level. "People stare down at a phone or up at a computer screen, and they squint without even realizing it," says facialist Nichola Joss of London's Sanctuary Spa. "Changing those angles eases the tension in your forehead immediately."

2. Rub your temples. If you're reading or working for long periods of time, take a 10-second break every 30 minutes to apply gentle pressure with two forefingers near the hairline; then, move the fingers in small, inward circles. This will help relieve tension and return your face to a neutral expression.

Pick the Right Cream

"A retinol cream is the gold standard when it comes to building collagen, which is what helps soften fine lines," says Patricia Wexler, MD, associate clinical professor of dermatology at Mount Sinai School of Medicine. But if you find retinol to be too harsh, consider creams containing peptides or ceramides—they stimulate collagen in a gentler way. "Just keep in mind that all collagen builders take a month of diligent use before you notice results," she says. A few more specifics on how to work these ingredients into your regimen:

THE DAYTIME FIX

Look for a multitasking, SPF-infused moisturizer with retinol and hyaluronic acid, which is a potent hydrator to help plump and replenish skin. **TRY: Neutrogena Rapid Wrinkle Repair Moisturizer SPF 30** ($18.69; *7yearsyounger.com/shop*) But not everyone can tolerate retinols. (See: Ask the Experts: What's Retinol?, p. 70). So if you're just starting out,

Exercise.

"It's not just what you're putting on your skin that matters," says Dr. Downie. "In my experience, patients who exercise regularly have better circulation, which gives them more of a natural glow."

you might want to begin with a nighttime retinol treatment (see *below*), and use a day cream with peptides or ceramides instead. These ingredients are also key if you already know your skin can't handle retinol. **TRY: Elizabeth Arden Ceramide Lift and Firm Day Cream Broad Spectrum Sunscreen SPF 30** ($47.49; *7yearsyounger.com/shop*). For both types of products, use a quarter-size amount *before* applying makeup.

THE NIGHTTIME FIX

Collagen builders do their best work at night, when your skin naturally repairs itself. So before bed, use a pea-size amount of an anti-aging night cream that contains retinol. **TRY: RoC Retinol Correxion Sensitive Night Cream** ($16.99; *7yearsyounger.com/shop*)—

ASK THE EXPERTS

Should I Try an Instant Wrinkle Smoother?

These products promise to immediately make fine lines look softer or less apparent for several hours without interfering with makeup. But do they work? According to Good Housekeeping Research Institute tests, yes (but only temporarily). And lucky for you, they do their best smoothing on forehead furrows! "I was wowed by them," says Birnur K. Aral, PhD, the Institute's Health, Beauty and Environmental Sciences Director. Look for ingredients like GABA, which relaxes muscle contractions, or oat-kernel extract, which provides lift by forming a film over skin. Apply in the morning—after serum, but before moisturizer and makeup. Results last up to 8 hours. **TRY: Skyn Iceland Angelica Line Smoother** ($65 for 1.5 oz; *7yearsyounger.com/shop*), which is a cream with GABA ("I was skeptical, but it really made a difference," said one tester).

Good Housekeeping Research Institute testers say it performed well for wrinkle reduction over eight weeks, especially on the forehead. If you need to go the retinol-free route, squeeze out a dime-size squirt of a formula that contains peptides. **TRY: Olay Regenerist Night Recovery Cream** ($17.86; *7yearsyounger.com/shop*). Once you apply either cream, allow it to be absorbed into your skin for a few minutes before bedtime, so it doesn't come off on your pillowcase. If you have problems with irritation from the retinol, try layering a plain moisturizer over your night cream, which could have a soothing effect.

MINI-MAKEOVER #4
Get Rid of Redness

Get this: One study from researchers in Austria and Germany shows that skin tone can add or subtract as much as 20 years to a woman's age! And while an uneven complexion can be caused by a variety of factors, one of the issues women struggle with most as they get older is redness. For some, that ruddiness develops as UV rays thin out skin and dilate or break the blood vessels near the surface. "This often happens to fair-skinned women first, because they soak up more sun damage more quickly over the years," says Dr. Graf. For others, it's a flare-up of the skin condition called rosacea. Even if you never really knew you had it, experts say its symptoms—which include persistent flushing and pimple-like bumps—are often intensified by sun exposure and age.

BONUS HAIR FIX
Get Some Strategic Fringe

Bangs can be better than Botox, say stylists—if you do 'em right. (See: Try Bangs, p. 56.)

Even Out Texture and Tone

Geller says the most nagging redness-related issue is the rougher texture that often comes along with it—this is especially true in cases of rosacea, she adds. So what's the solution? You want to create a fresh canvas with primer and foundation *before* you strategically cover up redness. Here's exactly how to do it:

1 **Start with a clear under-makeup primer.** "Primer allows makeup to float on the skin, rather than penetrate it, plus it resurfaces the skin if you've got bumps from rosacea." **TRY: L'Oréal Paris RevitaLift Miracle Blur Instant Skin Smoother and Finishing Cream** ($14.43; *7yearsyounger.com/shop*) or **Laura Geller Beauty Spackle Under Make-Up Primer** ($27.95; *7yearsyounger.com/shop*).

2 **Sheer foundations or CC creams won't cover redness well**, so you need formulas that are more opaque and provide extra coverage, says Geller. Rub the foundation between your fingers first, then apply—blending for even coverage. **TRY: MAC Full Coverage Foundation** ($31; *maccosmetics.com*).

3 **Now, look at your skin: Do you still see redness?** Spot-treat those areas with a thicker concealer (one that comes in a pot rather than a tube will usually do the trick). Take a little, put it on the back of your hand, and rub it around to warm it up. Then, use your finger to pat it lightly over foundation wherever you see red spots. **TRY: NYX Cosmetics Concealer Jar** ($4.99; *7yearsyounger.com/shop*).

4 **Use a lightweight, oil-absorbing finishing powder** to set concealer and foundation into place. A gentle dusting with a brush should do, says Geller. **TRY: e.l.f. Studio High Definition Powder** ($5.99; *7yearsyounger.com/shop*).

5 **Finally, add blush.** "Women worry it will bring out red tones, but your primer and foundation have created a second skin," assures Geller. Pale to medium skintones should use a soft pink or soft berry; for dark skin, go for a deeper shade of berry or rose. **TRY: Pür Minerals Château Cheeks Pressed Powder Blush** ($18; *purminerals.com*).

Ease Irritation and Soothe Inflammation

Reactive redness (caused by irritation), aging-related redness (caused by broken blood vessels) and rosacea (which is hereditary) can all be treated similarly, says Dr. Graf. So start with an SPF (sunlight makes redness worse, and red skin is often more sensitive to the sun), then use this dermatologist-approved checklist to find relief.

- **Prevent irritation.** "There are a lot of people out there who may be overdoing it with exfoliation or their anti-aging regimen," says Dr. Tanzi. "So it might not even be broken capillaries at all—it could just be chronic irritation." Try decreasing exfoliation to once a week or only using complex anti-aging treatments once a

Save Money on Anti-Aging Skincare

1. Cleanser Skip pricey options loaded with fancy anti-aging ingredients: Face wash doesn't stay on skin long enough to have much benefit. Your best bet is a basic non-soap cleanser—it's budget-friendly and gentler on skin, especially when you're using other anti-aging treatments. **TRY: Cetaphil Gentle Skin Cleanser** ($14; *7yearsyounger.com/shop*).

2. Toner This type of lotion was originally created to help balance skin's pH after the use of harsh cleanser. But there's no need for it when you use a gentle face wash. Sure, it will remove excess oil if you're especially greasy, but don't expect a big anti-aging boost.

day, and if you've seen a flare-up recently, ask yourself if you've added any new products to your regimen. Is the answer yes? It might not be the right product or ingredient for you, says Dr. Tanzi.

- **Try redness-fighting ingredients.** Once those capillaries near the surface of the skin are broken, there's not much you can do to fix them, short of in-office pulse-light treatments, says Dr. Graf. (Those run from $300 to $500 per session; you typically need three.) However, you can keep them from progressing—and lessen redness—simply by tweaking your skincare routine. Products formulated for sensitive skin are gentler and can reduce irritation, but there are also anti-aging ingredients to look for (found in many "anti-redness" or "redness-fighting" lines). Look for caffeine, licorice or white or green tea extracts. **TRY: Eucerin Redness Relief Daily Perfecting Lotion** ($15; at drugstores).

- **Rule out rosacea.** If you have rosacea, many of the ingredients mentioned above will help reduce redness and soothe skin, but your dermatologist may be able to prescribe something stronger as a long-term treatment, which is typically covered by insurance.

MINI-MAKEOVER #5
Make Sun Damage Disappear

Has the skin on your face gone from slightly freckled to blotchy and mottled? Starting in your mid-30s, sun exposure can send pigment-producing skin cells into overdrive, resulting in dark marks—known as age spots or sunspots. "Women who are fair or Asian are the most susceptible," says Valerie Callender, MD, an associate professor of dermatology at Howard University College of Medicine in Washington, DC. Other times, revved-up cells cluster together and cause melasma, which creates brown or blue-gray patches believed to be linked to estrogen: "It's more common in women with darker skin, women on birth control pills and pregnant women," says Amy Lewis, MD, an assistant clinical professor of dermatology at Yale University School of Medicine. The bottom line: Almost every woman will start seeing spots by the time she's in her 40s. But the good news is, a few simple makeup tricks and treatments can even you out and keep you clear.

Hide Spots the Right Way

The problem, Geller says, is that most women try to conceal dark spots *first*. "You get up, you look in the mirror, and you see that nagging hyperpigmentation on the side of your face—so you take your concealer and try to cover it," she says. "Then, when you apply your foundation—especially if it's a liquid or cream—you are basically wiping your concealer right back off." So instead, follow her easy steps to effectively neutralize darkness—and create an even skin tone all over:

1 **Apply your preferred foundation as you normally would.** "These spots are flat, so texture isn't as critical here," says Geller. (However, if you have all-over hyperpigmentation—not just a few

Improve melasma.
Experts say a series of
three to five in-office
chemical peels ($150
to $250 or more each)
can improve skin. Just
remember: If you shell
out that kind of cash,
you can't forget the
sunscreen—ever! You'll
be back to square one.

spots—you may need a weightier base that contains
more pigment. Mix it with a little moisturizer so it
goes on soft and smooth.)

2 Next, use a heavier concealer (ones
that comes in a pot rather than a tube are
typically thicker) about a shade lighter than your
foundation; peach undertones will help cancel out
brown. Pat it on top of dark spots using your finger.
TRY: NYX Cosmetics Concealer Jar ($4.99;
7yearsyounger.com/shop).

3 With a concealer brush (it'll give you more control), blend the
edges out, then set your makeup with a lightweight finishing powder
in the same color as your natural skin tone. You can also use it for
touch-ups throughout the day if darkness shows through. **TRY: e.l.f.
Studio High Definition Powder** ($5.99; *7yearsyounger.com/shop*).

Protect, Prevent and Lighten Up Dark Patches

Ready to fade those spots for good? Here's everything you
need to know, broken down into two straightforward steps:

STEP ONE: Protect and prevent.

First and foremost, your best line of defense is to prevent age spots in the
first place. Sunscreen is crucial. "If you're prone to spots, even a small
amount of sun exposure can bring them on," Dr. Callender cautions.
Same goes for melasma: No matter what you do to remedy it, those
blotches will recur if you're not careful. "I've seen patients spend
hundreds of dollars on melasma treatments (See: Quick Tip, *above*), then
they go to the beach without sunscreen, and boom, it's back," she adds.

So slather on broad-spectrum SPF 30 or higher every single day. (See: Save Face!, p. 67) Then, when you're outdoors, reapply on spots or melasma once an hour and any time your face gets wet. "Carry a sunscreen stick so you can swipe it often," says Dr. Lewis. Or, to keep your makeup intact, a mineral sunscreen powder is another great option. **TRY: Yes to Cucumbers Soothing Natural Sunscreen Stick SPF 30** ($8.97; *7yearsyounger.com/shop*) or **Brush On Block by Susan Posnick** ($30; *brushonblock.com*).

STEP TWO: Lighten up.

Now it's time to clear up the spots you already have. Here's how to tweak your skincare routine:

- **To fade sunspots away:** Use a serum or cream that contains retinol, says Dr. Callender. This powerhouse ingredient will shed your speckled skin and push new, healthy cells to the surface. **TRY: Dr. Dennis Gross Skincare Ferulic Acid + Retinol Brightening Solution** ($85; *7yearsyounger.com/shop*) or **Philosophy Help Me Retinol Night Treatment** ($45; *7yearsyounger.com/shop*). But if retinol irritates your skin, "pick a product with either alpha hydroxy acids or vitamin C," says Dr. Callender. Some common alpha hydroxy acids to look for in the ingredients list: lactic acid, citric acid or glycolic acid. **TRY: Physicians Formula Dark Spot Corrector & Skin Brightener** ($18.98; *7yearsyounger.com/shop*)—it contains lactic acid or **Jasön C-Effects Hyper-C Serum** ($34.38; *Jason-personalcare.com*), formulated with the most effective form of vitamin C.

- **To get rid of dark patches:** Anyone with melasma knows that it's very difficult to eliminate, and even doctors don't know exactly why. Many dermatologists stand by prescription hydroquinone as one of the most effective treatments, but with the controversy over its possible link to cancer, plus reports that when used incorrectly it can make pigmentation *worse*, some women prefer a product that contains kojic acid, glycolic acid, soy or retinol, all of which can help if applied every day. **TRY: Aveeno Positively Radiant Intensive Night Cream** ($14.97; *7yearsyounger.com/shop*) or **100% Pure Brightening Night Balm** ($32; *7yearsyounger.com/shop*).

MINI-MAKEOVER #6
Shrink Visible Pores

According to dermatologists, large pores are one of the most universal skin complaints. "My patients are obsessed with shrinking their pores," says Dr. Downie. "But if your parents had bigger pores, then you might also. It's mostly genetic." Sun damage and age will dilate them too, so you're not imagining it—they probably are looking larger these days. "Your collagen and elastin are disintegrating," explains Dr. Tanzi. "So we're basically losing the structural support that keeps them tight."

 ### Prime and Powder

Foundation can seep into pores, making them look obvious, while an oily surface can serve to magnify them further. So the trick of the trade, says Geller, is to use a good primer to create a silky barrier between your skin and makeup, then finish it all off with an oil-absorbing matte powder that reflects and blurs pores' appearance. The result is instant smoothness—and makeup that stays put all day! Your must-have products:

- **Under-Makeup Primer:** Choose one that's silicone-based, which glides on easily to create what Geller calls a "second-skin finish."

TRY: Boots No7 Stay Perfect Primer ($9.99; *7yearsyounger. com/shop*).

- **Oil-Free Foundation:** It'll keep skin looking soft and smooth. **TRY: Clinique Stay Matte Oil-Free Makeup** ($23; *clinique.com*).

- **Finishing Powder:** Here you want an ultra-lightweight, clear, matte product that's formulated to absorb oil and stop shine. **TRY: Pür Minerals Balancing Act Oil Control Powder** ($25; *pürminerals.com*).

Cleanse and Exfoliate

The only permanent solution for visible pores is a pricey in-office treatment using lasers, but caring for your skin can help lessen their appearance: For one, sweat and makeup may clog and stretch pores, making them appear more obvious, says Heidi Waldorf, MD, a New York City dermatologist. So to remove all that gunk and pore-dilating dead skin, switch to a daily cleanser with the exfoliators alpha hydroxy acid or salicylic acid. **TRY: Neutrogena Pore Refining Daily Cleanser** ($12.97; *7yearsyounger.com/ shop*). You might also consider investing in a vibrating brush, especially if your skin can't handle a harsher cleanser— paired with a gentle face wash, many patients feel it deeply power-cleans pores to dislocate dirt, says Paul Frank, MD, a cosmetic dermatologist in New York City. **TRY: Clarisonic Mia Sonic Skin Cleansing System** ($119; *7yearsyounger.com/shop*).

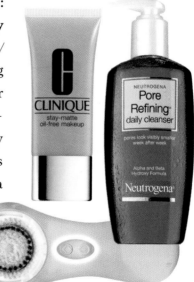

MINI-MAKEOVER #7
Remove Unwanted Hair

Thanks to genetics, some women (especially those with darker skin) are more prone to facial hair, while others never notice a single strand. But as you move into perimenopause—which can happen anywhere from your mid-40s to mid-50s—changing hormone levels leave you more susceptible to hair growth on your upper lip, chin and cheeks. Before perimenopause, hormones could be to blame for whiskers or fuzz too, but it's likely not a natural shift. See your doctor, who can rule out underlying health conditions, like polycystic ovarian syndrome.

 ### Remove Hair Safely

When it comes to ridding your face of pesky peach fuzz and unwanted hairs, there are lots of options—but what works best where? We talked to dermatologists and hair removal experts to put together this foolproof hair removal guide.

For peach fuzz on your cheeks

If hairs are especially long, you can trim them with scissors, says Dr. Graf. Otherwise, you're best leaving that fuzz alone. But because makeup can make those hairs more noticeable, a few tweaks to your morning routine can help hide them. Choose creamy foundations and blushes instead of powders, which can sit on top of fuzz like dust, and blend makeup in the direction hair is growing—this will help push hairs down.

For noticeable hair on your upper lip

Waxing is the safest and most effective solution, says Sasha Belousova, a hair removal expert at Paul Labrecque Salon and Spa in New York City. It only needs to be done every four weeks, and it's gentler on skin than depilatory creams. If you can't afford to see a pro regularly (an upper lip wax costs anywhere from $8 to $12, on average) or simply prefer to do it at home, follow these tips to minimize irritation:

1 **To prepare, be sure to stop using topical anti-aging products 72 hours prior to waxing.** Ingredients like alpha hydroxy acid or retinols make skin more sensitive.

2 **Purchase a kit that includes both pre-size strips and finishing wipes that remove wax.** (But if you just buy strips, baby oil also works to get the wax off.) **TRY: Veet Ready-to-Use Wax Strips for Bikini, Underarm and Face** ($8.99; at Walmart).

3 **Clean skin thoroughly first.** Then carefully follow the instructions on your kit, but remember: Always pull it off against the hair growth. That means doing each side separately, removing the strip toward the nose.

4 **Afterward, soothe skin with a gentle gel** or cream containing aloe vera, or if you have sensitive skin, apply a hydrocortisone cream, which will reduce irritation and redness.

For dark, wiry strands on your chin:

The consensus here was overwhelming, among doctors and aestheticians alike: Don't pluck! "I see too many women who irritate the skin with tweezers or who get ingrown hairs," says Dr. Downie. If you just have a few strays, your best bet is to carefully trim these wiry whiskers with facial hair scissors once or twice a week. Otherwise, get them tweezed by a pro, or try a depilatory cream—since it's usually such a small patch of skin, potential irritation is less traumatic—but still be *extra* careful. "These are tricky," says Dr. Graf. "Test a very, very small area first." Results will last about one to two weeks. **TRY: Olay Facial Hair Removal Duo** ($24; at drugstores).

 ## Consider Laser Removal or Electrolysis

If facial hair is a serious source of stress, you may want to consider investing in electrolysis or laser hair removal from a board-certified doctor, which are your only permanent hair removal options. Just be advised: Lasers (you'll need three or more sessions at about $150 to $200 a pop) will only hit thick, dark hairs, and "electrolysis takes a long, long, long time," says Dr. Downie. Electrolysis treatments last between 15 minutes and 1 hour, and the number of appointments needed varies from person to person—but you'll probably need to go back multiple times over the course of at least one year. Both treatments can also be painful, although many doctors will apply a topical anesthetic to dull the discomfort.

The Quickie Guide to a Great Face

If you do nothing else, try one or all of these tips to refresh your face.

1. Apply an SPF Moisturizer This is two-fold: You're protecting yourself from irritating sun damage and infusing your face with skin-plumping moisture, which instantly gives you a dewy sheen and makes lines look less pronounced.

2. Even More Sun Protection Dermatologists beg you to invest in a hat! Because there are some UV rays that can permeate sunscreen, when you're outside for long periods of time, the more extensive the protection—the better.

3. The Right Foundation The proper base layer for your makeup is increasingly crucial as you age: It's not just tone you have to worry about anymore, but also texture.

4. Lots of Water...Lots! It will hydrate your skin from the inside out, and drinking more water will also take the place of caffeine—and sugar-laced beverages, which can zap your skin of its radiance and speed up the aging process.

5. Embrace Blush Every top-notch makeup expert says that, when done right, it's the secret to shaving off years. Why? Blush doesn't just brighten your face, but lifts it too!

6. Repair Overnight Now that you know what anti-aging ingredients are best for you, use them, at least at night. Skin repairs itself as you snooze, so whatever you apply will be more effective

7. Exfoliate Weekly Cell turnover slows as you get older, which means you need to slough off those dead skin cells. (It'll help with almost everything—from restoring your natural glow to fading sunspots!)

Brighten Your Eyes 3

How to banish bags, conceal every crease and instantly look less tired

Mini-Makeover #1
Soften Crow's Feet
Lessen the appearance of fine lines around the eyes
95

Mini-Makeover #2
Diminish Dark Circles
Conceal and dampen down shadows for good
99

Mini-Makeover #3
Nix Bags and Puffiness
Diffuse and disguise swelling so your face looks refreshed
104

Mini-Makeover #4
Smooth Out Crepey Lids
Even out crinkly eyelids and apply makeup the right way
107

Mini-Makeover #5
Lift Droopy Lids
Sculpt brows to combat sagging
112

Mini-Makeover #6
Give Sunken Eyes Shape
Create definition in just a few easy steps
112

Mini-Makeover 7
Open Tired Eyes Wider
Create emphasist to look wide awake–always
113

Mini-Makeover #8
Create Face-Framing Brows
Give them shape (and fill them in) to shave off years
114

Mini-Makeover #9
Get Lusher Lashes
Boost length and volume to make eyes pop
117

"If your eyes still look at life with wonder, then you will seem young." — *Goldie Hawn*

When it comes to your eyes, the signs of aging don't appear overnight—but it can seem like they do—and this highly expressive area is the first place most of us notice the signs of aging. "Much of it is genetics, but the skin around the eyes tends to be one of the thinnest spots on the face, meaning it's easy to damage," says Paul Frank, MD, a cosmetic dermatologist in New York City. "And it is also an area that many women have neglected over the years."

While you've likely spent a lot of time applying mascara or perfecting your everyday look, how often did you take a cotton swab and apply SPF to your entire lid? What about those times you scrubbed off all of your foundation, but were too exhausted to remove every bit of eyeliner?

It's OK. In fact, the great news is, you can make your eyes look bigger and brighter—and even give them a lift—in mere minutes. Just as your eyes can instantly age you, giving them the proper daily care—and learning a few tricks from the best makeup artists in the business—will shave years off your appearance. "For the same reasons that the skin around the eyes is more susceptible to damage over time, it is also potentially more susceptible to making improvements," says Dr. Frank.

MINI-MAKEOVER #1
Soften Crow's Feet

Those little wrinkles that branch out from the corner of your eyes? First of all, be proud of them! They're a sign of years and years of happy times. "This area sees lots of movement when we smile and laugh," says Elizabeth Tanzi, MD, a dermatologist in Washington, DC, who adds that squinting in the sun is another major culprit here. "Eventually, as the skin ages, it loses its snap-back quality. That's when the crow's feet start to appear."

 Soften and Deflect

There's an insider secret to lessening the appearance of crow's feet and other fine lines around the eyes—and it goes beyond simply sealing off creases or covering up wrinkles. If you really want to make these lines less noticeable, "draw attention to the center of your lids with a touch of shimmer shadow," says makeup artist Jordy Poon. And a "winged" or cat-eye look, where eyeliner extends out past the end of the lid, is not helping. Instead of giving you a lift, it's just going to settle into your wrinkles, making them more pronounced. Here's your step-by-step tutorial, which will hide those tiny creases and give your eyes a wider, brighter look right away.

1 Prime your skin. Before putting on makeup, particularly for a special occasion, use a facial primer that fills in wrinkles to create a smoother canvas. Bonus: It also helps makeup last longer! **TRY: L'Oréal Paris Revitalift Miracle Blur Instant Skin Smoother and Finishing Cream** ($14.43; *7yearsyounger.com/shop*).

2 **Reflect light.** Dab a liquid highlighter that's close to your skin tone on top of crow's feet; blend outward. This will reflect light away from imperfections while giving the illusion of an even complexion. **TRY: Boots No7 Skin Illuminator** ($9.99; *7yearsyounger.com/shop*).

3 **Line your eye.** Use a brown or black pencil to line your top lids, being careful not to extend past the corner. **TRY: CoverGirl Perfect Blend Eye Pencil** ($5; *7yearsyounger.com/shop*).

4 **Lay down a shadow base.** Swipe a nude or pale gray matte shadow all over your lids, then put on mascara. **TRY: Revlon ColorStay ShadowLinks in Bone or Greige** ($2.99 each; *ulta.com*).

5 **Add some shimmer.** Pat a subtle champagne shimmer shadow (for dark skin, go gold) on just the center of your lid. **TRY: Revlon ColorStay ShadowLinks in Gold** ($2.99; *ulta.com*).

FIX IT SO IT LASTS

Protect and Repair

You can't completely reverse these little lines once they appear, but preventing further sun damage—and keeping this delicate area well-hydrated with a collagen-stimulating eye cream—will help plump up the skin and soften the wrinkles' appearance, says Dr. Tanzi. Here's your two-step approach.

STEP ONE: Protect.

- **Start with an SPF** of at least 30 every day, making sure to cover the delicate area around your eyes. This helps protect your skin from UV rays that break down collagen and cause wrinkles. Dr. Frank recommends using a cotton swab to apply your regular facial sunscreen or moisturizer with SPF to your eyelids—that way it won't get rubbed into your eyes—but you might also want to consider a product specifically formulated for this area. "If it doesn't say eyes on the bottle or box, look for a mineral sunscreen made with zinc oxide," says Jeanette Graf, MD, a dermatologist in New York City. They're typically chemical-free and adhere better to your skin, which will prevent any running or stinging. (And don't worry: These formulas are carefully blended, so they won't leave a blue-white cast, like pure zinc-oxide paste.) **TRY: Colorscience Sunforgettable Loose Mineral Eyescreen SPF** 30 ($18; *7yearsyounger.com/shop*).

- **Toss on sunglasses** any time you go outside, especially between 10 A.M. and 4 P.M.—even if it's just bright, not sunny! It will stop those automatic squinting movements that deepen crow's feet, while also blocking both UVB and UVA rays. "Sunscreen does a great job with UVB," says Dr. Tanzi, "but even the best sunscreens might let some UVA rays through." (To choose the best sun-protective, age-appropriate frames, See: Fashion Fix, p. 98.)

STEP TWO: Repair.

The advice here is simple: You want to gently apply a good moisturizing eye cream to clean skin twice a day, in the morning and night, says Dr. Tanzi. Part of the power of these products is that they hydrate and smooth the skin, making wrinkles look less pronounced. But the second layer of magic comes from ingredients that help strengthen and repair skin long-term—just be patient. "Once you find one you like, you've got to give it four to six weeks to see lasting results," says Dr. Frank.

- **Choose It:** Creams with retinols (See: What's Retinol?, p. 70) will reduce wrinkles by bumping up collagen production and decreasing its breakdown. **TRY: Neutrogena Rapid Wrinkle Repair Eye Cream** ($16; *7yearsyounger.com/shop*). That said, retinols can be harsh on the delicate skin around your eyes, so you might want to try a product with peptides, which have the same effect but tend to be a bit milder, according to Dr. Tanzi. **TRY: Avon Anew Clinical**

FASHION FIX
Frame Your Face

The frames you pick are just as important as the lenses. "Most sunglasses are good at blocking out the UVA and UVB rays," says Dr. Tanzi. "It's usually just the shape you need to worry about—and the bigger the better!" Larger frames mean larger lenses, which translate into better protection of the delicate skin around the eyes and less squinting, which deepens crow's feet. But can you really pull it off? Yes, says *Woman's Day* Style Editor Donna Duarte-Ladd. "Sunglasses are the ultimate coverup. Large frames come in all shapes, so fit yourself with the right one to complement your style." Follow this easy guide:

If your face is...	Choose
Round (full cheeks + rounded jawline)	Square or wide rectangular shades
Oblong (long face, narrow cheeks + chin)	Wrap or oversize shades
Heart-shaped (square forehead + jawline)	Cat's eye or round shades
Square (square forehead + jawline)	Round or oval shades

Pro Line Eraser Eye Treatment with A-F33 ($13.95; *7years younger.com/shop*) or **Perricone MD Hypoallergenic Firming Eye Cream** ($56; *7yearsyounger.com/shop*), which improved fine lines by 29 percent in Good Housekeeping Institute lab tests.

● **Apply It:** Tap on eye cream with your ring finger (tugging at this fragile skin can cause sagging, and your ring finger is your weakest, so it has the softest touch). Start below the inner corners of your eyes, and pat along the ocular bone to the outer corners.

MINI-MAKEOVER #2
Diminish Dark Circles

If you're plagued by pesky undereye circles, the biggest culprit here is genetics. Some women are simply born with fair or thin skin and less fat in this area, which can cause capillaries and veins to show through—especially when blood pools there because of lack of sleep, says Joshua Zeichner, MD, a dermatologist in New York City. "Those people typically have little blue-tinged dark circles, even since they were young," he says. "But as skin loses collagen and thins further, they become even more pronounced." Chronic inflammation, like from allergies, can also shine through—giving skin a brownish tinge.

 Cover Up Darkness

Many women with dark circles under their eyes try to hide them with too much concealer, which just draws more attention to the area by creating a pasty effect. But carefully applying a small amount of the right product will give your face a flawless, even appearance without looking caked on, says Mally Roncal, a celebrity makeup artist and founder of Mally Beauty Cosmetics. Follow these easy steps:

1 Apply eye cream, which should be at least SPF 30, first.

2 No matter what your skin color, choose a creamy concealer with a yellow undertone; it'll counteract undereye shadows by masking blue tones. Apply with a brush for extra precision, so that you can target only the dark area. (To blend, don't rub it in. Instead, press it in gently with your ring finger.)

3 Set your concealer with a dusting of powder that matches your skin tone (bonus if it has a little radiance to brighten this area).

HABIT REHAB
Keep Eyes Looking Fresh

Are you guilty of bad habits that aggravate your eyes and add to a swollen, puffy appearance? Turn them around, so you wake up bright-eyed, and stay that way.

1. **Remove eye makeup...** no matter what! Keep a jar of makeup remover pads next to your bed for nights when you're too tired to wash your face. Bonus: Some now come with ingredients like cucumber, chamomile and caffeine, which will cut down on puffiness too. **TRY: Almay Soothing and Depuffing Gentle Eye Makeup Remover Pads** ($5.99 for 80; at drugstores).

2. **Don't rub your eyes.** It's an easy way to catch an infection that makes your eyes red and irritated, and friction aggravates inflammation, making dark circles more noticeable, says Jeanine Downie, MD, a dermatologist in Montclair, NJ.

FIX IT SO IT LASTS

Erase the Darkness

There's no at-home treatment that's going to banish your circles forever, says Dr. Zeichner, but there *are* some strategic products you can add to your daily regimen to help lessen their appearance. The ingredients you look for are going to depend on the shade of your circles:

- **Blue-tinged:** This means they're likely the result of swollen blood vessels near the skin's surface, so go for a caffeinated formula in the morning. "Caffeine constricts blood vessels," says Dr. Zeichner. **TRY: Origins No Puffery Cooling Roll-On for Puffy Eyes** ($25; *origins.com*).

- **Brown:** It's probably a hyperpigmentation issue. "The body responds to inflammation—from things like allergies and rubbing—as an injury, sending extra melanin to repair it," says Dr. Zeichner. Here, the superstar eye brightener ingredients are vitamin C (**TRY: Clinique Even Better Eyes Dark Circle Corrector**, $24.95, *7yearsyounger.com/shop*) and niacinamide (**TRY: CoverGirl+ Olay Eye Rehab CC Cream**, $9.29, at drugstores), used morning or night.

TRY: Your Best Undereye Products

- Creamy concealer: **e.l.f. Essential Cover Everything Concealer in Corrective Yellow** ($2; *eyeslipsface.com*)

- Concealer brush: **Sonia Kashuk Core Tools Concealer Brush** ($5.99; at Target stores)

- Powder: **bareMinerals Illuminating Mineral Veil** Finishing Powder ($13; *7yearsyounger.com/shop*)

7 YEARS YOUNGER MAKEOVER
The Problem: Tired Eyes

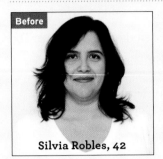

Before

Silvia Robles, 42

With three children under 8 years old, Silvia—whose husband travels frequently for work—worried that juggling the kids on her own was running her ragged. "Sometimes I look older because I'm so worn out," she said. "I wish I had more energy." Silvia has also watched her weight steadily creep upward, until she realized she was carrying an extra 25 pounds. "That was the sign that I have to start making myself a priority too," she says.

THE FIX:

- **Expose Your Eyes:** Stylist Nunzio Saviano, of the Nunzio Saviano Salon, gave Silvia a chin-length bob. This helped to remove dry, split ends. When styling her hair, Saviano blew hair away from her face at the roots to give her hair more movement. (See: Try a Youth-Boosting Style, p. 48.)

- **Avoid Heavy Makeup:** Rather than spread on thick foundation, makeup artist Sue Pike applied a light tinted moisturizer first, then camouflaged Silvia's undereye issues by blending concealer on top. "Less is more—otherwise you just draw more attention to that area," she says. (See: Cover Up Darkness, p. 99.)

FINISHING TOUCHES

1. Use Highlighter on Eyes: A sweep of light-diffusing powder just below the brow bone and along the inner corners instantly wakes up eyes.

2. Apply Raspberry Lipgloss: Putting on a bright lip shade helped draw attention away from Silvia's dark circles.

3. Wear Jewel Tones: Silvia discovered that jewel-toned clothes (like this blouse) could make the whites of her eyes look brighter.

Reduce puffy lids.
Brew a cup of
caffeinated black tea
using two tea bags.
They contain tannins,
a natural diuretic to
help drain fluid. Place
the cooled down tea
bags over your eyes
for 10 minutes.

MINI-MAKEOVER #3
Nix Bags and Puffiness

Even in your teens or 20s, you probably had mornings where you woke up with tired, swollen eyes. Fluid tends to pool there while we sleep, and salty foods and alcohol can both trigger excess swelling. As we get older, though, the area under the eye can get extra puffy, thanks to a redistribution of fat. Dr. Zeichner explains it like this: "When you're young, this area is like a well-packed suitcase: Everything fits. But with age, the suitcase starts busting at the seams." These little fat pads are like sponges, adds Dr. Frank. "They don't just protrude on their own, but they also soak up fluid and swell."

 Diffuse and Disguise Swelling

For mornings when you're in a rush, start off with a de-puffing undereye cream or gel. "Many have caffeine, which temporarily dehydrates and shrinks fat cells," says Dr. Zeichner. Pick one that's oil-free, so makeup doesn't smear. **TRY: Garnier Skin Renew Anti-Puff Eye Roller** ($13; at drugstores). From there, you'll want to disguise bags

BONUS FOOD FIX
Bananas Banish Puffiness

A banana a day could help keep the eye bags away, says celebrity nutritionist Kimberly Snyder, author of *The Beauty Detox Foods*. "They're high in potassium, which helps regulate the fluid levels under your eyes."

with a good concealer—and choose makeup colors that play down redness and lid puffiness, rather than enhance it. Your step-by-step guide:

1. **Tap on concealer.** "Fat deposits typically appear yellowish under the skin," says Schlip, "so you want to go darker here to manipulate the light." Her rule of thumb: Pick a product that's the same shade as your skin or even one shade darker, and apply *only* to the padded, puffy part. Then, pat on your regular concealer (two shades lighter than skin tone) directly below that.

2. **Blend it.** Put a little BB cream, CC cream or tinted moisturizer (Not sure what these are? See: Find Your Best Base, p. 73) with an illuminating factor on your finger, then lightly pat it over the top of both concealers, to soften their appearance.

3. **Apply eye makeup.** To minimize redness, stick with eyeshadows or liners that are gray if you have fair or medium skin; for dark skin, go with navy. And be sure to curl your lashes and put on mascara, which will help hide swollen top lids. **TRY: L'Oréal Paris Silkissime Eyeliner by Infallible in Charcoal and Plum** ($7 each; at drugstores).

Reduce Inflammation

Only surgery can get rid of fatty deposits permanently. But for chronic puffiness, dermatologists and facialists agree— this is one case where some simple habit changes and a few pampering DIY treatments can help soothe skin and reduce swelling overall. Here's how to rehab your routine:

- **Every night:** Sleep with two pillows under your head, so any fluid around your eyes can drain, says Shirley Chi, MD, a Los Angeles dermatologist. Also try to avoid triggers like salty foods or red wine, which is loaded with skin-bloating sulfates.

● **In the morning:** On days when swelling is especially bad and you have 10 extra minutes to spare, this retro fix still holds water: Place cucumber slices in the freezer before you get in the shower. After your shower, lie down with your head propped up on two pillows and place the cold cucumbers on your eyes. "The cold closes down the blood vessels in the area, giving you temporary relief," says Dr. Frank.

● **Once or twice a week:** Give yourself a DIY spa treatment before bed using tea, which is a great natural anti-inflammatory. Here, a three-step guide from Robin Berger, lead therapist at Cornelia Spa in New York City.

1. Steep two chamomile tea bags, then let them cool to room temperature.

2. Next, lie back with your head elevated. Place a tea bag over each eye for 10 minutes, then rinse your face with cool water.

3. Follow with this 5-second massage: Holding two fingers together, pat a dot of eye cream under each eye, working from the inner corner out. With each pat, gently push the skin toward your temple. "It helps move the excess fluid out from under your eyes."

MINI-MAKEOVER #4
Smooth Out Crepey Lids

As you get into your late 30s and early 40s, it's common to start to see a bit of wrinkly skin on your eyelids, and eventually, it might even feel a bit slack. What's happening here? "The eyelid skin is very thin and delicate to begin with," says Dr. Tanzi, "plus it tends to dry out easily." Over the years, this double-whammy takes its toll on the fragile area, a process accelerated by sun damage. Far too often, Dr. Frank warns, women neglect applying SPF to this area for fear of irritating the eyes.

 Play Down Lids and Play Up Lashes

Whether it's a shimmery shadow or a too-heavy eyeliner pencil, certain types of makeup can accentuate crinkly lids. So the key to masking crepiness is to use products with the right texture—ones that will glide over and flatten those miniscule creases. Then, "you can easily deflect from wrinkly eyelids just by emphasizing your lashes," says Poon. Here's your easy how-to:

1 Start with a makeup primer. It will even out skin, which helps your eye makeup last longer, and it also prevents shadow from creasing, says Poon. Spread it on gently with fingertips. **TRY: L'Oréal Paris RevitaLift Miracle Blur Instant Skin Smoother and Finishing Cream** ($14.43; *7yearsyounger.com/shop*) or **Laura Geller Beauty Spackle Under Make-Up Primer** ($27.95; *7yearsyounger.com/shop*).

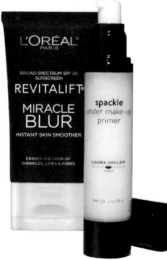

2 Apply a matte shadow. Shimmery shadows enhance crepiness, but a matte shadow will flatten an eyelid with lots of texture. Sweep a warm taupe (use brown on dark skin) on lids, up to the creases. **TRY: Revlon ColorStay ShadowLinks in Bone or Greige** ($2.99 each; *ulta.com*).

3 Line your top lids. Use a black marker eyeliner (for fair skin, try brown or navy), since the lightweight formula glides over delicate skin and won't creep into wrinkles. To apply, draw a thick line just above your lashes, starting at the outer corner and ending just short of the inner corner. **TRY: Maybelline New York EyeStudio Master Precise Ink Pen Eyeliner** ($5.99; *7yearsyounger.com/shop*).

4 Brighten the line. With a small shadow brush, trace a gleamy eyeshadow in the same color (think: satiny, not shimmery) over the liner.

5 Accentuate lashes. Finish with two coats of volume-enhancing mascara. **TRY: L'Oréal Paris Voluminous Butterfly Mascara** ($7; *7yearsyounger.com/shop*).

Protect, Hydrate, Repair

"Crepey eyelids are everyone's nemesis after a certain age!" says Ellen Marmur, MD, a dermatologist in New York City. But a few simple tweaks to your routine ("hydration here is key," she adds) can help to moisturize and smooth.

- **Cleanse carefully.** Use gentle cleansers, if anything, says Dr. Marmur: "Sometimes I just put a drop of face lotion on a good old baby wipe to remove residual eye makeup." Otherwise, look for something oil- or cream-based. **TRY: Philosophy Purity Made**

Simple One-Step Facial Cleanser ($36 for 16 oz; *7yearsyounger.com/shop*).

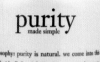

- **Moisturize with eye cream.** A specially formulated but gentle anti-aging eye product is important for smoothing and rejuvenating your skin here. "They are less likely to cause irritation, redness or stinging so you can actually use them twice daily," says Dr. Marmur. Massage it gently over the eyelids and underneath the eye in a circular motion with your ring finger. **TRY: Mario Badescu Hyaluronic Eye Cream** ($18; *7years younger.com/shop*).

- **Watch your habits.** "Get at least seven hours of sleep; don't eat salty foods after 5 P.M. or go for the second glass of booze; and exercise first thing in the morning," says Dr. Marmur. "These tips are for fluid balance, which will help to reduce the visibility of lax eyelid skin."

Make Eyes Bigger and Brighter

Do you feel like your eyes no longer pop? Your eyes sink back some as you age, which allows more of the lid to hang down, making your eyes seem smaller. What's more: The skin on your brow bones can also start to droop at the outer corners, creating a tired, hooded look. Why is it happening? Chalk it all up to the same loss of elasticity and structure that's causing lids to look crinkly and skin to sag elsewhere, says Dr. Zeichner. That means the best advice for lasting skin repair is the same as issues like crow's feet and crepiness—you want to protect the eye area from further

The Problem: Sunken Eyes

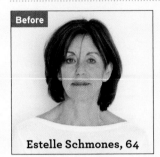

Before

Estelle Schmones, 64

Even though she's technically retired from her teaching job, Estelle still runs all over town as a private tutor for elementary school students— and she keeps up with the 30-somethings in her kickboxing class. "I'm a young kind of 64," says the brand-new grandma. "But even though I exercise a lot and eat well, I know there's no way to completely stop the changes I see in my face—that's why I would love to learn a few techniques to help me look as young as I feel."

THE FIX:

- **Prime First:** The Laura Geller makeup team applied a makeup primer around Estelle's eyes and across her lids to ensure all the eye makeup would go on smoothly and not sink into fine lines. It also helped give her lax skin a tighter appearance. (See: Smooth Out Crepey Eyelids, p. 107.)
- **Give Lids a Lift:** Geller's team used two tiny tricks to open up Estelle's eyes. First, a sculpted brow with a high arch helps draw the eye up (See: Lift Droopy Lids, p. 112). Then line the upper lashes, making sure it's a little thicker—and ticks up—at the outer corner of her eyes (See: Give Sunken Eyes Shape, p. 112).

FINISHING TOUCHES

1. Make Cheeks Glow: A sweep of youth-boosting pink blush to the apples of Estelle's cheeks helped make her complexion pop.

2. Line Lips: Her smile was lined with a nude-colored lip pencil to give the color staying-power and prevent it from feathering.

3. Try Hoop Earrings: Adding a fun accessory helped distract attention away from her eyes. They also evoke youth without being too young.

66

*My eyes
look so
much more
open!"*
–Estelle

damage with an SPF and sunglasses, and use a collagen-stimulating eye cream twice a day (see Protect and Repair, p. 96). However, your makeup approach may differ depending on the issue you struggle with most, so we've broken it down into three easy, targeted, fast-fix solutions.

MINI-MAKEOVER #5
Lift Droopy Lids

Fear not: "When skin on the lid and under the brow becomes less taut, there are creative ways to draw less attention to the area," says pro makeup artist Laura Geller. Her best and easiest trick? Sculpt your brows, as a well-defined arch will draw the eye up, giving your lids an instant lift. (For easy advice on how to groom your brows and give them a natural-looking fill, See: Create Face-Framing Brows, p. 114.)

MINI-MAKEOVER #6
Give Sunken Eyes Shape

Hooded, sunken eyes lose definition, so the key here, says Geller, is to line them—on top and bottom. "Women often skip the upper lid when it's hooded because they think you can't see it," says Geller. "But darkening the lash lines on top and bottom will bring back the shape where it has softened—so your eyes pop." Use a dark pencil (black, dark brown or charcoal all work), and follow these simple tips:

- **Start thin; get thicker.** On both the top and bottom, begin at your first lash in the inner corner, and draw a thin, firm line that gets slightly thicker as you approach the outer corner. A felt or gel liner will offer more precision, but "the real trick is to walk it across in small little doses—don't try to swipe one line right across the lid."

- **Connect the upper and lower lids.** Line the bottom last, then tick it up at the end, so it connects with the top. This creates an almond shape that looks bigger and wider, says Geller.

MINI-MAKEOVER #7
Open Tired Eyes Wider

Even if you're not using liner to create a wider shape, one fast and easy way to perk up your eyes is to strategically emphasize them at each end. Here's how to do it:

- **Give your lashes extra oomph.** Simply curl them for 10 seconds before applying a black volumizing mascara; then, use a second

BONUS FASHION FIX
Make Your Eyes Pop

Wearing clothes in the right shades brings out your eye color, which makes eyes look instantly wider, brighter and younger, says *Woman's Day* style editor Donna Duarte-Ladd. And while jewel tones flatter everyone's faces, this chart can help you pick an outfit that emphasizes your eyes, according to color.

If your eyes are...	Wear:
Blue	Any shade of blue will bring out the blue in your eyes.
Green	Go for blue with green tones (like aqua or teal) or deep green.
Hazel	Emphasize the lighter flecks in your eyes with earth tones and deep chocolates.
Brown	Deep crimsons, purples or burgundy will draw out brown's richness.

QUICK TIP

Get extra lift. Brush a highlighting shadow (a light color like bone, beige or eggshell) directly underneath the eyebrow, says Taymour. It'll highlight the brow bone and accentuate the arch, for a face-lifting effect.

or third coat on *just* the outer corners. This will open up the eyes and make them appear wider.

● **Highlight the inner corners.** Finish off your eye makeup routine by using a sponge-tip applicator to apply a highlighting powder or light eyeshadow (bone or eggshell with a little shimmer work best) to the inner corners of your eyes. The bridge of your nose typically casts a shadow here, but this trick reflects light instead, so eyes look bigger and brighter.

MINI-MAKEOVER #8
Create Face-Framing Brows

So your brows are suddenly a little sparse, or maybe there are bald spots here and there? "This is mostly genetic, but it also has to do with your habits over the years—plucking, waxing, etc," says Dr. Frank. You might notice thinness in some places, and long, wiry hairs elsewhere, says Taymour Hallal, a brow specialist at Paul Labrecque Salon and Spa in New York City. Every woman is different, but putting down the tweezers for a month can help you figure out where hair is gone for good—or how you might be able to reshape around the thinness. (One note: If you notice an unusual amount of hair loss at the outer edge of your brows, so that they appear shorter than they've always been, or hair stops growing toward your temple, tell your doc. It could be a sign of a thyroid condition.)

Give Brows a Face-Framing Fill

Almost any makeup artist will tell you that a well-defined brow is not only easy to achieve, but that it's a secret anti-aging weapon—maybe even more important than good foundation! This tutorial from Mally Roncal will help you create a natural-looking eyebrow with makeup—one that will open up your eyes, frame your face, and sharpen your features.

1 Comb your brows into shape with an old mascara brush (clean it first with alcohol), then use a pencil to make light, feathery strokes throughout (not just in the thin spots). Go one shade lighter than your natural brow color; if you're blonde or gray, use a taupe color. **TRY: Maybelline New York EyeStudio Master Shape Brow Pencil** ($6.49; *7yearsyounger.com/shop*)—it has a brush built in, so you don't even need an old mascara wand.

2 Next, switch to a brow powder. Using both is key: Pencil alone is too harsh, but powder by itself is too wimpy. Gently sweep the powder—in the same color as your pencil—over your brows (most come with a small stiff, angled brush). **TRY: Laura Mercier Brow Powder Duo** ($22; *7yearsyounger.com/shop*).

3 Finish by misting hairspray on your mascara brush, and combing your brows one last time. This blends the pencil and powder together for a soft, believable look.

Shape for Enduring Fullness

If you want to take years off your look by reshaping your brows, it could help to make an appointment with a good brow specialist at a salon, says Taymour. (Costs typically range from $15 to

QUICK TIP

Skip lotion. As you grow brows in, don't put lotion on top of the area—it can clog hair follicles. "My clients can't believe how much faster their brows grow once they stop doing this," says Sania Vucetaj, owner of Sania's Brow Bar in New York City. "Some say that hairs that haven't grown in for years suddenly reappear."

$40 per appointment, depending on the method and your location.) "I have a client who calls me Taytox because she jokes her brows are better than Botox!" he says. "That's the effect that you can get by picking the right shape." After you let brows grow in for at least a month, a specialist can carve the right arch by waxing, tweezing or threading. Then, you can maintain it on your own. A couple of quick basics, if you're trying it at home:

1 Pluck, don't wax. Tweezing is the most precise way to shape your own brows. Waxing without a professional can traumatize that delicate skin as you get older, leading to crepiness.

2 Trim before you tweeze. Maybe you used to pluck any longer hairs that grew out beyond your ideal brow line, but now you might need them there for fullness. If they originate within your brow's shape, don't pluck. Just trim them down to keep them in line, says Taymour.

3 Create balance. Follow your natural brow shape, then sculpt it to complement your face. If your face is more angular, do a soft curve. For a rounder face, a more defined arch, which will sharpen your bone struc-

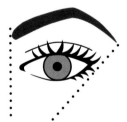

ture. **Tip:** Use a pencil to determine where brows should start (hold it straight up, parallel to the bridge of your nose) and end (line it up diagonally from the bottom corner of your nose and past the outer corner of your eye).

MINI-MAKEOVER #9
Get Lusher Lashes

Have you noticed that your once-thick lashes are a little shorter or less voluminous than they used to be, even when you swipe on a layer or two of mascara? It's the same story as your disappearing brows: A mix of genes and past damage (from things like careless curling or constant rubbing) might cause them to thin out or to not grow quite as long as they used to, says Dr. Frank. "Any sort of chronic trauma to the hair follicle adds up, until eventually that follicle doesn't grow a hair anymore," he says. The answer, then, is a mix of simple makeup magic and mistake management—because being a bit more cautious about the bad habits that damage follicles will protect *and* preserve the lashes you have.

 Create Lots of Volume!

Luckily, restoring a dark lash line and adding thickness and curl won't just give you the appearance of fuller lashes—but it will also open and lift the eye tremendously. Follow this simple how-to from celebrity makeup artist Mally Roncal.

1 Start by curling the top lashes. (If you don't do it, you might as well not wear mascara at all, she says.) The trick is to do it carefully, so you don't tug lashes or damage the hair follicle. No repeated pulses; just squeeze once at the base and hold for a few seconds. **TRY: Shu Uemura Eyelash Curler** ($20; *shuuemura-usa.com*).

2 Dot black eye pencil between lashes, applying from underneath. Then blend it with a liner brush.

3 Smush your mascara wand right in your lash base, wiggle it a few times slowly, then pull it through, lifting it up and toward your nose. This trick will make your eyes look more open.

4 Next, hold the wand vertically and gently skim it across your lashes in a windshield-wiper motion. This fans them out and gets rid of any clumps on the tips.

5 Mascara on your bottom lashes finishes the look, so hold the brush vertically and lightly paint each lash. That way, it won't smudge. If you suffer from dark circles, though, you might want to skip this step—playing up your lower lashes could just draw attention to any undereye shadows.

TRY: The Best Big-Volume Mascaras

Almost every makeup artist we talked to recommended using black mascara. "One swipe of a good black will give you the fullness of four swipes of brown, without crumbling or smudging or irritating your eyes," says Schlip. What's more: The fewer the coats, the less weight you'll put on delicate lashes, keeping them strong and healthy. A few of our favorites:

- **L'Oréal Paris Voluminous Butterfly Mascara** ($7; *7yearsyounger.com/shop*)

- **Maybelline New York Volum'Express The Falsies Big Eyes Mascara** ($8.69; *7yearsyounger.com/shop*)

- **CoverGirl Bombshell Volume Mascara by Lashblast** ($9.59; *drugstores.com*)

FIX IT SO IT LASTS

Preserve What You've Got

Lashes are certainly one of the areas of your face where makeup can work absolute wonders, and hopefully, that promise is enough to temper this little tidbit of truth: Once you lose them or see significant thinning, there's not much you can do to get them to grow back faster, longer or thicker. (Your only option to that effect is a pricey prescription serum called Latisse. See: Ask The Experts—What's Latisse?, p. 120.) Still, with some prudence and special care, you can protect the lashes you have. In fact, by keeping them strong and healthy enough to grow to their full length—and fixing the habits that cause additional breakage or shedding—your eyelashes might look more lush in a matter of weeks. Here's your lash-care checklist:

- **Don't rub your eyes.** Whether it's from chronic allergies, sleep deprivation or just plain old habit, many women are forever rubbing their eyes. Here and there, it won't hurt, "but it's very much like sun damage—over time, it adds up," says Dr. Frank. So if you do it, you've likely done it for decades; now's the time to stop pronto to prevent pulling out those already weakened hairs.

- **Always, always, always remove eye makeup.** The longer mascara is caked on, the more it will harden and weigh down your lashes—and eventually, those heavy hairs can crack under the stress, especially if you're putting added pressure on them as you sleep. So never go to bed without thoroughly removing all eye makeup. And of course, when you go to take it off, be sure to do so gently. Soak a flat cotton pad in makeup remover (you only need an oil-based one if your mascara is waterproof), then hold it on your eye. "The key is to give it one, two, three seconds, instead of just rubbing," says Geller. "That extended but gentle contact will make it dissolve—then you can just lightly wipe it away."

● **Curl to 10—and release.** A lash curler is an unbelievable tool to have in your arsenal—it adds oomph, lifting and opening up even the smallest, most tired of eyes. But because the lash root is so extremely delicate, you need to curl with the utmost care. Just press together and hold for 10 seconds, then release—never pull or yank.

ASK THE EXPERTS

What's Latisse—and Should I Try It?

Latisse is the brand name for a prescription medication called *bimatoprost*, and it is currently the only FDA-approved treatment to enhance lashes. You apply it to your lash line with a tiny applicator twice daily. (According to the results of its company-sponsored product trials, it can double fullness in 16 weeks.) Every dermatologist we talked to raved about Latisse, so if thinning lashes are your issue, yes, you might want to try it. But there are a few things you need to know first. There have been some reports that Latisse can change your eye color, although Dr. Frank says that risk is mostly for those with green eyes—and very tiny on top of that (less than 2 percent). According to Dr. Frank, it'll probably cost you about $60 a month to start. "Because it works so well, most people use it twice daily for a few months, then maintain a few times a week after that." (At that point, he estimates the cost to be about $20 per month.) If you're considering this treatment—it could also work on thinning eyebrows—talk to a dermatologist, who can help you figure out if it's right for you.

The Quickie Guide to Beautiful Eyes

If you do nothing else, try one or all of these tips for younger-looking eyes.

1. Don't Forget SPF! The delicate skin around your eyes is especially susceptible to sun damage that can speed up the appearance of crow's feet and crinkly lids. So carefully apply sunscreen daily—use a cotton swab if you're afraid of irritating your eyes.

2. Begin and End Your Day With Eye Cream Look for collagen-stimulating retinols or peptides and hydrating ingredients (like hyaluronic acid or glycerin); they'll work together to smooth, plump and repair skin for short- and long-term benefits.

3. Sunglasses On...Always. When outdoors (regardless of season!) this is a good move for two reasons: You block the UVA rays that SPF can't completely shut out and you stop squinting, which deepens crow's feet.

4. Get Sounder, Smarter Sleep Nothing makes eyes look older and more tired than actually being tired. Prop your head up on a pillow and snooze for at least 7 hours to help reduce fluid buildup that causes bags and circles too.

5. Primer First You don't have to use makeup to cover crow's feet or crinkly lids, but if you do, invest in a primer. It'll create a smooth surface, so that powders, foundations or shadows don't accentuate tiny ripples.

6. Give Brows a Quick Fill Accentuating your eyebrows with a pencil or powder is a must! They frame your face, which opens up your eyes and sharpens your other features.

7. Boost Your Lashes Giving them a quick curl (10 seconds) and adding a coat of a black mascara is one of the easiest, fastest ways to lift your lids and make your eyes pop.

Boost Your Smile 4

Plump up lips, whiten teeth and smooth out fine lines.

BOOST YOUR SMILE

66 Smiling is one of the best beauty remedies." *– Rashida Jones*

Experts say that grinning wide is a natural drug. When you smile, your brain releases feel-good chemicals, which can relax your body, giving you an allover glow. It's a fact: "When people see a big, bright smile, they see instant youth," says Emmanuel Layliev, DDS, a cosmetic dentist in New York City.

But that's exactly why the little signs of aging in and around the mouth can be such a downer. Whether you're worried about deepening laugh lines or afraid to show off stained teeth, these tiny problems cause a hit to your overall confidence. And even if you didn't smoke or bake in the sun when you were younger (the two biggest behavior-related aging accelerators in this area, which could make wrinkles crop up as early as 30), genetics will still cause some subtle changes as you enter your 40s. "The lip thins, plus years and years of natural habits, like sipping through a straw or laughing or enunciating, lead to the appearance of fine lines," says Jeanette Graf, MD, a dermatologist in New York City.

Luckily, there are ways to get your smile confidence back—and then some. In this chapter, you'll get easy advice from top dermatologists, sought-after cosmetic dentists and in-demand makeup artists.

MINI-MAKEOVER #1
Soften Dry, Cracked Lips

Every woman has battled chapped lips, especially during winter. That's exactly why, when it comes to your smile, one of the first aging-related changes you may see—dry lips—is something you might not even associate with age at all. But as you grow older and your skin loses its moisture, your lips are at a unique disadvantage: They have a thin epidermal layer that always produced very little oil to begin with, plus—as the gateway to your mouth—they've taken quite a bit of abuse over the years. "Just from years of brushing our teeth, eating, drinking, licking our lips and being outdoors in the sun, the skin gets damaged—even from speaking!" says Dr. Graf. "There's a lot of movement in the lips, but not much moisture. So many women start to notice a dryer, rougher surface all year round."

Making sure lips are hydrated isn't just the key to eliminating dryness, though. It's also the number-one, most crucial step for preventing or masking other lip-related signs of aging—little mouth lines, loss of color, disappearing volume. "Keeping moisture on your lips is very, very, important, and the thicker the product, the better," says Dr. Graf. The simple truth: A mouth that's dry is going to look more wrinkled than it actually is. So here's how to hydrate and smooth parched lips, for an instantly younger-looking smile—and also things you can do to nourish and repair lips for good.

FIX IT FAST **Moisturize and Smooth in the Morning**
When lips are rough and flaky, you need to focus first on plumping and softening with a good balm, says celebrity makeup artist Melanie Mills. From there, it's all about choosing the right conditioning lipstick—one that's brightening but weightless, so that it glides easily over a rougher surface.

STEP ONE: Moisturize.

Start with a rich balm that has at least SPF 15, or higher. Lips lack melanin and are especially susceptible to sunburn, which will dry and chap them further. Look for ingredients like vitamin E and shea butter, and apply it first, before you even moisturize your face. That way, you can let it settle in while you do the rest of your makeup. "When lips are properly moisturized and smooth, the color will apply seamlessly," says celebrity makeup artist Sonia Kashuk. **TRY: Sun Bum SPF30 Coconut Lip Balm** ($4; *7yearsyounger.com/shop*).

STEP TWO: Add color.

Your go-to lipstick might be adding to the dryness problem: Anything matte will zap moisture, as will "long-lasting" products that contain alcohols. "They really, really dry out the lips," says Mills. "It's time to

TRY: Your Best Moisturizing Lipsticks

- A conditioning tinted lip gloss/balm: **Almay's Color + Care Liquid Lip Balm** ($5.99; at drugstores)

- A good vitamin-enriched lipstick: **CoverGirl Continuous Color Lipstick** ($6.49; at drugstores)

- A long-lasting but moisturizing formula: **Boots No7 Stay Perfect Lipstick** ($10; *Target.com*)—Women in Good Housekeeping Institute tests found it lasted over 3 hours, and were fans of its creamy texture, which left their lips feeling smooth.

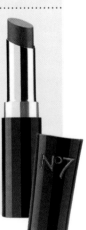

give them up—at least for regular, everyday wear."

Fortunately, there is a wide selection of moisturizing lipsticks, stains and glosses on the market that are specially formulated to soften and smooth. Most will tell you so, but if not, just look for ingredients like shea butter, palm oil, vitamin E or glycerin on the label. As for choosing a color, "very pale or very bold lip colors will make a dry mouth look even more scaly, so stick with soft, natural shades like rose or, for darker skin, a subtle, reddish berry," says Rebecca Restrepo, global makeup artist for Elizabeth Arden.

 ### Repair Lips Overnight

Wake up to soft, supple lips! Apply a moisturizer before bed so it has 8 hours to work its magic.

- **If they're just a little dry:** Try an ointment with active ingredients including petrolatum or glycerin. **TRY: Aquaphor Healing Ointment** ($13.89 for 14 oz; *7yearsyounger.com/shop*)

- **If they're cracked or chapped:** Look for a specially formulated overnight ointment that contains a mix of potent healing ingredients, such as shea butter, lanolin, glycerin, beeswax and/or vitamin E. However, you don't want "medicated" balms that contain tingly ingredients like camphor, menthol, eucalyptus and peppermint oil: "Their cooling effect may feel good, but sometimes they can further irritate chapped lips," says cosmetic chemist Ni'Kita Wilson, CEO and director of innovation at Catalyst Cosmetic Development, which develops products for skincare and beauty brands. **TRY: Aquaphor Lip Repair** ($3.97 for .35 oz; *7yearsyounger.com/shop*) or **Neosporin Lip Health Overnight Renewal Therapy** ($4.30; *7yearsyounger.com/shop*).

MINI-MAKEOVER #2
Plump Up Thinning Lips

Your once-lush lips might look less plump. "Even if you were to avoid the sun our whole lives, you start to lose volume in your lips and your mouths around 40," says Dr. Graf. Plus, the color of your lips might soften and bleed a little at the top, leading to a skinnier, duller, less-defined look. What's the cause? Blame it mostly on sun damage and your body's diminishing ability to stimulate the growth of collagen, which is what gives your lips their plumpness and structure.

BONUS FOOD FIX
Eat for Smoother Lips

Severely chapped lips can be a sign of nutritional deficiency. If you're constantly suffering, see your doctor. That said, certain foods can help. Try these picks from Kristin Kirkpatrick, MS, RD, LN, at the Cleveland Clinic Wellness Institute.

- **Eggs:** All animal products have B_{12}, a nutrient that can keep lips from cracking, but eggs also pack a dose of anti-inflammatory choline.

- **Broccoli:** This green vegetable is high in B_2 (also known as riboflavin), a vitamin that may help ward off chapped lips.

- **Avocado:** This fruit's healthy fats are the superstar ingredient for nourishing your hair and skin (lips included!) from the inside out.

FIX IT FAST **Plump and Brighten**

Here's some great news: The lips are one of the easiest areas of the face to make over, says Kashuk. Temporary plumpers can work to restore some fullness (See: Ask the Experts—What About Lip Plumpers?, p. 130), but the right combination of lipstick and liner—along with a few easy application tricks—will give your lips an all-day roundness and richness that shaves years off your face. Here's how to do it:

1 **First, make sure the lips are moisturized.** A good, hydrating balm won't just soften and plump lips, but it should help your makeup last longer too.

2 **Next, blend just a little bit of foundation over the lip and lip line** to "fill those very fine lines and give you a more even surface to work on," says Kashuk. Then, use a small eyeshadow brush to apply a bit of brightening powder to the bow of the lip, as well as just around the end of the upper lip line. "It's going to reflect light, giving your lips a lift," she says. **TRY: Sonia Kashuk Brightening Powder** ($10.39; at Target stores).

3 **Now, take a lip liner pencil that matches your lipstick color and use it to shape your lips.** For your upper lip, start at one corner and come outside your natural lip line ever so slightly—lifting up, *then* rounding out to the bow. "When you start at the bow, you tend to stick too close to your lip line, for a harsher effect," says Kashuk. Repeat on the other side. **TRY: Wet n Wild Color Icon LinerLip** ($1.50; at drugstores).

4 **Fill in your lips with the liner pencil to give them a longer-lasting base,** then use your finger to lightly trace the color around the edges. This will create a softer, more natural looking line.

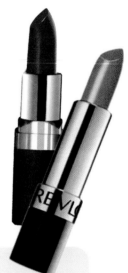

5 **Finally, apply your lip color** (See: Pick the Right Lipstick, p. 136). "Matte lipsticks are too flat, but satin finishes are a middle ground," says Kashuk. For brightness, add a dab of gloss in the middle of the lips, to avoid bleeding. **TRY: Revlon Super Lustrous Shine Lipstick** ($6.99; *7yearsyounger.com/shop*) or **Rimmel London Moisture Renew Lipstick** ($5.47; *7yearsyounger.com/shop*).

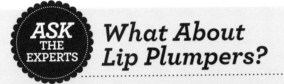

ASK THE EXPERTS

What About Lip Plumpers?

There are now *tons* of products—from base coats to actual glosses—that claim to plump your lips. Do they work? Absolutely, says Dr. Graf, although the results are temporary (usually a couple of hours). "They cause a reaction in the skin that makes it plump," she explains. "The tingle can be alarming—but they're harmless." The only problem is, plumping products can vary greatly. Some can be thick or sticky, others might dry out your lips or cause actual stinging pain—not just the slight tingle you're told to expect. You may need to experiment to find one you like, but once you do, you can apply a clear formula as a base (**TRY: Physicians Formula Plump Potion Needle-Free Lip Plumping Cocktail, Clear Potion** ($10.34; *7yearsyounger.com/shop*) or swipe a tinted one (**TRY: Too Faced Lip Injection Color Bomb! Moisture Plumping Lip Tint** ($21; *sephora.com*) across the center of each lip like a gloss, as described in Step 5, *above*. Discontinue if lips get dry or scaly; irritation and lack of moisture—no matter what the cause—can speed up aging.

FIX IT SO IT LASTS

Protect, Hydrate, Repair

The only immediate but longer-lasting solution for thinning lips is an injectable filler, like Restylane and Juvederm. (It costs about $600 per syringe—most patients require one or two—every six months.) But you don't necessarily need fillers. By protecting lips from the sun, keeping them moisturized and applying a collagen-stimulating treatment, you can create fuller, younger-looking lips, says Dr. Graf.

- **Every morning:** Dryness highlights thin lips, so use a lip moisturizer with hydrating ingredients like vitamin E or shea butter, as well as SPF 30, since sun also speeds up thinning. "Don't just use regular lotion on your lips," says Ellen Marmur, MD, a cosmetic dermatologist in New York City. "Hydrating lip balms are waxier, so they really stick to the skin and continue to deliver moisture." You might also want to consider making your daily lipstick one that comes formulated with peptides, which can stimulate collagen production over time. **TRY: Elizabeth Arden Ceramide Ultra Lipstick** ($16.99; *7yearsyounger.com/shop*).

- **Every night:** Most anti-aging lip treatments are formulated to smooth and soften, but ingredients like hyaluronic acid, peptides, retinols or phytoestrogens can boost collagen production, adding fullness and firmness over time. Slather it on at night and let it work its magic. **TRY: Veneffect Anti-Aging Lip Treatment** ($85; at Neiman Marcus stores). When the Good Housekeeping Research Institute put lip treatments to the test, the Veneffect formula won out for making lips appear plumper after four weeks. "It made my lips feel soft and smooth and appear fuller," said one tester. The active ingredient: phytoestrogens, which are plant-based compounds thought to help rebuild skin.

7 YEARS YOUNGER MAKEOVER
The Problem: Thin Lips

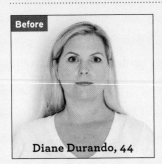

Before

Diane Durando, 44

"I'm a work in progress, and I think sometimes that work can get halted," says Diane, mom to two young kids who just started her own business and takes care of her disabled father. She has been following the *7 Years Younger Anti-Aging Plan* since its inception— mostly to help her stress less, eat better and sleep more. Now Diane is eager to learn how to apply her makeup to help her look younger.

THE FIX:

- **Minimize Redness:** The Laura Geller Makeup team applied a clear makeup primer before a more opaque foundation to help even out both the texture and tone of Diane's skin—a big issue for her ruddy complexion. (See: Even Out Texture and Tone, p. 80.)

- **Bigger, Brighter Lips:** Instead of Diane's go-to neutral lipstick with a matte finish, Laura Geller's pros put on a brighter rosy hue with a hint of shimmer. The light reflecting particles will help give the illusion of a fuller pout. (See: Plump Up Thinning Lips, p. 128.)

FINISHING TOUCHES

1. Get Long Layers: The stylist added long, face framing layers to give her thick, heavy hair more bounce but kept the length.

2. Use Concealer Around Lips: To help plump and define, Geller's team used a dab of concealer around her mouth (not on lips) and blended it in.

3. Apply Clear Lipgloss: A touch of shiny gloss to the center of both the top and bottom lips helped make Diane's pout appear to be larger.

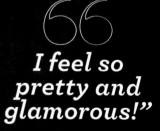

> ❝ *I feel so pretty and glamorous!"*
> –Diane

MINI-MAKEOVER #3
Smooth Out Little Lip Lines

As you get older, the first wrinkles around your lips will likely be the perioral lines—they're those itty-bitty, super-fine, vertical crinkles on and along the upper lip. "There can be a huge variation as to when these begin to appear, depending on your habits," says Dr. Graf. "But some women will start to see them in their late 30s and early 40s."

So what's causing these wrinkles, which—without the right care—will increase in depth and number over time? Your skin loses fat and retains less moisture in its lower layers; as a result, it's less plump—and you see crinkling on the surface. At the same time, you're also losing elasticity. "When we're younger, the skin just snapped back to its original form," says Elizabeth Tanzi, MD, a dermatologist in Washington, DC. "But now every time you pucker up or drink through a straw or smoke, it etches those lines in a little bit deeper."

 ### Prime and Pump Up Lips

When it comes to concealing these creases with makeup, the challenge here is two-fold. First off, without the right technique, your lipstick can seep inside your lip lines, highlighting the wrinkles and giving your mouth a rougher, more textured appearance. But your lip lines can also cause your lipstick to bleed—so you need to be able to contain the color and make it last. Sound daunting? Not when there's one simple solution: lip primer. Just follow this easy tutorial from celebrity makeup artist Joanna Schlip for a more even but radiant color that sticks:

1 **Start off with a good, hydrating daily face cream with SPF,** and be sure to swipe over your lips. (If your lips are extra dry, use a hydrating balm with a waxy texture.) Moisture will immediately plump and soften lips, making creases and wrinkles less noticeable.

2 **To prevent feathering, strategically fill in lip lines with a moisturizing nude lip primer.** Work a little less than a pea-size dollop between your index finger and thumb, then apply a sheer coat, patting it along the edge of the lips. Allow to dry for 30 seconds. "Less is more, so don't put it everywhere if you don't need it," says Schlip. "The more of your skin's natural radiance that can show through, the better." **TRY: e.l.f. Studio Lip Prime & Plumper** ($3; *eyeslipsface.com*).

3 **Finish off with a sheer but dense liquid lipstick in a universally flattering color, like watermelon or poppy.** "The color is strong, but not cakey, so lips will look moist, smooth and healthy," says Schlip. **TRY: Stila Cosmetics Stay All Day Liquid Lipstick in Fiore** ($22; *7yearsyounger.com/shop*).

TRY: Fresh Sugar Lip Treatment SPF 15

This smoothing and softening stick was the indisputable favorite in Good Housekeeping Research Institute's tests of anti-aging lip treatments, and it earned extra raves for its ability to minimize fine lines on and around the lips after a month's use. (The active ingredient: sea fennel, a plant peptide believed to smooth and repair fine lines and wrinkles.) Just be sure to store it in a cool place—its consistency can get very soft in the heat, say testers. ($25; *7yearsyounger.com/shop*)

Pick the Right Lipstick

Lipstick is tricky: The proper color can make you look years younger, while certain shades or textures will age you considerably. There's a sweet spot, though, say makeup artists—and here's how to find it.

- **Your skin tone.** It's by no means a hard and fast rule, but a **peachy or coral shade** is ideal for yellowish or olive skin, while berries look great on dark skin—and a rosy pink works on just about everyone, says celebrity makeup artist Mally Roncal.

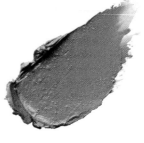

- **Your age.** When you're in your 30s, you can get away with everything, from shiny glosses to flat mattes. As you enter your 40s, however, you need more moisture and less shimmer to lessen the effects of dryness and fine lines. "A thick lipstick will instantly age you," says Schlip. Her best suggestions for middle age and beyond: **satin finishes, liquid lipsticks** ("you don't have the thickness, but you still have the intensity"), and slightly glossy stains.

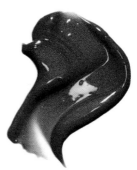

- **Your attitude—and the occasion**. "Listen, sometimes there are no rules about color!" says Kashuk, "It's about the confidence you carry when you wear it." While shades close to your natural lip color will give you the best full lip that sticks for all-day wear, **a brighter berry, a deeper-but-moisturizing mauve, or a bold red** can create an elegant nighttime look (think: a dinner date or wedding).

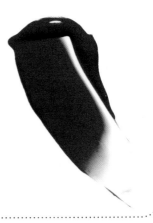

Moisturize and Repair

If lip lines are an issue, you might want to consider replacing your moisturizing lip balm or nighttime lip ointment with an anti-aging treatment that has a mix of stronger ingredients that correct and prevent collagen damage—like hyaluronic acid, peptides, retinols (See: What's Retinol?, p. 70) or phytoestrogens. You can apply it as much as you'd like, but at least, you'll want to use it in the morning and at night. (Just be sure to follow it up with a lip balm containing SPF in the A.M.)

HABIT REHAB
Let Your Mouth Relax

"If you're pursing your lips or sipping through a straw, you're reinforcing movements that create lip lines," says Dr. Graf. "Make those movements less pronounced and you'll relax those muscles just like Botox would—and that can help some pretty hard-core lip lines, too." Eliminate wrinkle-causing habits:

- **Stop smoking.** It doesn't just lead to a breakdown in collagen, but the repeated lip-pursing motion will carve little lip lines deeper and deeper.

- **Don't use straws.** Drinking lots of water? Great! Your skin needs to stay hydrated from the inside out. But if you've been using one of those reusable cups with the straw, switch it out for a bottle that lets you tip and sip. Other times (think: smoothies) drink straight from the glass.

- **Ditch gum.** "If you chew all day and keep the lower part of your face in constant motion, it increases the signs of aging there," says Karyn Grossman, MD, a dermatologist in Santa Monica, California. (Here's why: The repeated motion might weaken collagen in the skin around your mouth.) "I tell patients to switch to breath mints if they need an oral fix or fresh breath."

MINI-MAKEOVER #4
Lessen Deeper-Set Wrinkles

Along with those crinkly little lines on and around your upper lip, you might start to notice some deeper-set folds surrounding your mouth. The first are laugh lines (or, more technically, nasal labial folds), which run from your nose down to the corners of your mouth. The second are marionette lines, which etch out a path from the corners of your mouth down to your chin—kind of like the exaggerated lines you'd see on a ventriloquist's puppet.

When and how heavily these wrinkles appear depends largely on genetics, but they're mainly caused by movements (smiling, laughing, pouting, talking) that cause the skin to crease in the same place again and again. "Our skin just doesn't have the same elastic, snap-back property it had when we were younger," says Dr. Tanzi. What's more: Sun and smoking can further accelerate the damage that causes them to appear, making your habits—once again—key for prevention.

FIX IT FAST — **Smooth Out and Conceal Wrinkles**

To mask the appearance of deeper set creases around the mouth, like marionette lines and laugh lines, the real key is to avoid heavy foundations, which will settle into wrinkles, exaggerating their depth. "You can't really cover a wrinkle—there's no such thing!" says celebrity makeup artist Laura Geller. "You simply want to soften it and make it appear less sharp." Here's how to do it, from start to finish:

1 **Moisturize first with an SPF-formulated facial moisturizer and lip balm.** Dry skin always makes wrinkles look more pronounced.

2 Now, fill in wrinkles with a good face primer, dabbing it into each laugh line or marionette line. TRY: L'Oréal Paris RevitaLift Miracle Blur Instant Skin Smoother and Finishing Cream ($14.43; *7yearsyounger.com/shop*) or Laura Geller Spackle Under Make-Up Primer ($27.95; *7yearsyounger.com/shop*).

3 Next, take a lighter concealer into the depths of the line, and feather it out with your finger. This "trickery," as Geller calls it, will make the crease appear less steep. (You could also use a flesh-colored pencil to trace the line.)

4 Finish with a lightweight, moisturizing foundation—Geller recommends BB creams here. (Don't know what those are? See: Find Your Best Base, p. 73.) Here's why: A heavy foundation will cake and crease easily over wrinkled skin—primed or not. But if you need heavier coverage for other issues (like redness), you can use your same product, just be sure to blend it over those lines twice with a sponge. TRY: Physicians Formula Super BB All-in-1 Beauty Balm Cream ($10.90; *7yearsyounger.com/shop*).

Moisturize, Repair, Replenish

Once you have deep-set wrinkles, like laugh lines or marionette lines, you can't really erase them. (The only longer-term treatment, like with thinning lips and lip lines, is an injectable filler, such as Restalayne or Juvederm.) That said, you *can* make over your skincare regimen to hydrate the skin—giving it a plumper, wrinkle-filling effect—and stimulate collagen production, which will prevent those creases from deepening.

- **In the morning...try an anti-aging serum:** Serums are lightweight and easily absorbed into the skin, plus they're packed with a higher dose of active ingredients than plain facial moisturizers. So apply a pea-size amount before your SPF moisturizer—this will allow the serum to seep deep into the skin. (Allow at least eight weeks to start seeing results.) **TRY: Estée Lauder Perfectionist [CP+R] Wrinkle Lifting/ Firming Serum** ($89.99 for 1.7 oz; *7years younger.com/shop*)—it's on the pricey side, yes, but the Good Housekeeping Research Institute found it to be best for minimizing fine lines and wrinkles.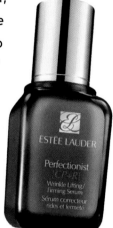

- **At night...replace plain moisturizer with a stronger night cream:** One with retinols will help diminish wrinkles, while also moisturizing and firming skin. If you know retinols irritate your skin, though, look for one with peptides instead. (They'll be more moisturizing for dry skin types, too.) (See: The Nighttime Fix, p. 78.)

- **Once a week...gently exfoliate to remove dead skin cells:** "When you have dead skin on your face, it can actually make the valleys of these wrinkles appear deeper," says Dr. Marmur. That's where exfoliating comes in. "Problem is, women often overdo it with chemical exfoliators, and they come in beet red, bumpy and inflamed." You can use your favorite product once a week, or try this gentle at-home method, which Dr. Marmur swears by:

1. Soak a washcloth in warm water.

2. Rub a teaspoon-size drop of facial lotion into it. (It doesn't need to be an expensive, specially formulated product, she says; any old lotion that won't irritate your face will do.)

3. Gently massage your face with it. "Not only are you removing skin cells that are ready to come off, but massaging will also dilate blood vessels to increase circulation—so you're just getting a really robust delivery of the rejuvenation proteins that your body already makes for you."

MINI-MAKEOVER #5
Brighten and Whiten Teeth

Many women may notice a yellow tint to their teeth in their 20s, whether it's because of twice-daily lattes or a smoking habit in high school and college. But with age, our mouths become even more susceptible to discoloration—yellowing, unfortunately, is almost inevitable. "Teeth are porous, so over time they're going to stain and darken," says Dr. Layliev. Even wine and juice can give them an off-white tinge.

What's really happening here, on *and* under the surface? Basic wear and tear—brushing, eating, drinking—erodes the tooth enamel, even in women with the best dental hygiene. Then acid from food or drink can permeate that barrier to punch little holes in the teeth, where stains settle in. Luckily, though, at-home bleaching *really* works if you give it time, say experts. "It's worth it," says Irwin Smigel, DDS, a cosmetic dentist in New York City. "If your teeth look white, you automatically look younger."

FIX IT FAST

Brighten Your Lips

The advice here is so easy, you won't even believe it: "If you put on a lipstick with yellow or orange undertones, you're accentuating the yellowness," says Kashuk. Paler shades that don't create any contrast against your teeth won't help your case either, she adds. So for an instant smile makeover? All you have to do is swap out that problem color for a bright hue that has a blue or purple tinge. Here's your guide:

- **If you usually wear an orange-y coral:** Try a berry pink, which will give a similar radiance and freshness, without the yellow undertones.

- **If you usually wear a tomato red:** Try a plum or a richer red with a purple tinge. It will create the same kind of contrast against your other facial features—but will bring out whiteness too.

ASK THE EXPERTS

I Think My Teeth Look Shorter—Am I Crazy?

No, you're not, says Dr. Layliev. As we get older, teeth wear down, the result of years of chewing, biting and grinding while we sleep. "Shorter top teeth can also cause your lips to sag inward, creating a thin tight-looking smile, he says, "instead of one that's fuller, softer and more youthful." The only way to fix short teeth permanently is to have your dentist elongate them with bonding or veneers (costs vary, depending on the extent of the work that needs to be done), but there are things you can do to prevent more deterioration. For one, don't chew on pens or pencils, and also consider asking your dentist about a custom night guard, which will prevent grinding. They can run anywhere from $400 to $750, but your dental insurance may cover a chunk—or all—of the cost. Plus, they can last for up to five years, making them a worthwhile investment over time.

- **If you usually wear a frosty pink:** Try a rose or mauve with a hint of blue tones. These colors are equally understated, but also add some brightness that boosts your smile.

FIX IT SO IT LASTS Bleach Teeth and Keep Them White

First, the bad news: All those whitening toothpastes and mouthwashes sitting in your medicine cabinet aren't going to make your teeth any whiter (they're just meant to *maintain* whiteness—more on that later). Still, experts all agree that at-home bleaching treatments can be highly effective, especially if your stains are yellow-tinged. "Those are the easiest to get rid of," says Dr. Layliev. Brown stains tend to be a little more stubborn, and grays are the most difficult of all to reverse; these colors may require an in-office treatment, he adds. From there, maintenance is critical (See: Habit Rehab, p. 146). Here's what you need to know.

The Basics on Bleaching at Home

Three groups of people shouldn't do their own whitening: those whose teeth are painfully sensitive to cold, anyone with crowns or fillings on their front teeth (they won't whiten and will end up looking much darker than surrounding teeth), and people whose enamel seems more gray than yellow (due to intrinsic stains from antibiotics like tetracycline taken in childhood). But if that's not you? You're in the clear to give at-home bleaching a try, say experts.

When it comes to whitening teeth, it's all about the length of time the peroxide comes in contact with your teeth—that's why toothpastes and rinses won't do much to lighten your smile. Over-the-counter kits that come with trays have the right idea, says Dr. Smigel, but because the carriers your teeth rest in aren't custom-fit, it could lead to uneven—or lackluster—results. Every single dentist we talked to recommends whitening strips for that reason: "The peroxide is fixed to the strip, which stays fixed to your teeth, without moving or rinsing out," says Dr. Layliev. "They really work the best." All you need is patience: Because the peroxide on the strips isn't highly concentrated, it will take a good three to five weeks of regular use to see results.

To maximize your whiteness and bleach safely at home, keep these three rules in mind:

1 **Time it right.** For best results, use an at-home whitener after a professional cleaning, says Dr. Layliev. Why? Bleach won't penetrate plaque. Even a thorough at-home brushing will help, but those with sensitive teeth may want to wait at least an hour before bleaching.

2 **Do a smile test.** When you're younger, you typically only have to bleach your top teeth—they're all that show when you smile. "But as we get older, the bottom lip starts to pull back and reveal our lower teeth," says Dr. Layliev. So look in the mirror and flash a big smile before you bleach. If you can see your bottom chompers, you may need to whiten them, too.

TRY: Crest 3D Whitestrips Professional Effects

These thin, flexible, gel-coated strips lightened teeth up to four shades (2.2 on average) in 20 days when applied to teeth as directed—once a day for 30 minutes, Good Housekeeping Research Institute tests showed. ($37.54; 7yearsyounger.com/shop).

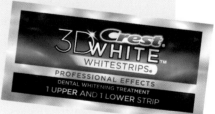

3 **Soothe sensitivity.** Tooth pain is a common side effect most people experience, typically for a day or two. Using a specially formulated toothpaste can help lessen it (**TRY: Sensodyne Pronamel Toothpaste for Sensitive Teeth**, $5.99; at drugstores), as can avoiding acidic foods and beverages (like grapefruit or orange juice) for up to a week after whitening.

What You Need to Know About In-Office Treatments:

If you're in a hurry or have gray stains, the type of bleaching done in your dentist's office is—without a doubt—your fastest and most effective option. It can lighten teeth 10 shades in just an hour, according to the American Academy of Cosmetic Dentistry (compared to two shades in 20 days for your best at-home option). "It's like an exfoliation process for your teeth," says Dr. Layliev. "The teeth are cleaned to remove the top layer of stain, then we actually extract the deeper stains from the pores using a peroxide gel under a high-intensity light." Exact methods and prices differ, but you can expect a three-cycle treatment to cost around $600. Depending on how well you take care of your teeth afterward (See: Habit Rehab, p. 146), that whiteness can last anywhere from one to five years. Most programs will also send you home with custom-fit trays for at-home follow up. With those stubborn gray tetracycline stains, for example, you'll need about two to three months of regular application to reach peak brightness.

BOOST YOUR SMILE

HABIT REHAB
Easy Ways to Keep Teeth White

Whether you're applying strips at home or seeing your dentist for a treatment, bleaching won't do any good if you still smoke or drink black coffee. Here's how to make sure your teeth stay white, bright and healthy.

Eating: Anything that's sticky and dark (like barbecue sauce) is going to cling to teeth when you eat it; if it's warm, it'll penetrate the surface too, causing even deeper stains. If you can't avoid such foods, chase each bite with water (whether sparkling or flat) and swish it around in your mouth for a few seconds to rinse away the residue, says Dr. Layliev. Also beware of colored candies, gums and popsicles—the types that turn your tongue purple or red. They can stain teeth too, if consumed regularly.

Drinking: Dark beverages bathe your mouth in tooth-tinting liquid, which is bad news for your whitened smile. (A good rule of thumb: If it would stain a white T-shirt, it will stain your teeth!) Switching from red wine to white wine helps, and having a piece of cheese beforehand can build a calcium barrier that protects teeth from tinting. As for coffee, you can sip it through a straw (suck without pursing, to avoid lip lines), or at least add milk. It acts as a buffer to coffee's tooth-eroding acid, which makes stains seep deeper.

Cleaning: Flossing directly after eating is important to remove residue. As for brushing, you'll want to wait about 30 minutes. "After we eat, the pH within the mouth is very acidic, and any type of normal brushing will erode enamel," says Dr. Layliev. That's where whitening toothpastes and mouthwashes come in—just make sure the rinse is color-free, dentists warn. They work like exfoliants, scrubbing stains from the surface before they have a chance to penetrate the tooth. Dr. Layliev likes the Dentisse line, which uses Kaolin clay as the active ingredient: "The paste has tested best in removing stains without over-abrading the enamel," he says. "But since it doesn't have fluoride, I'd use a regular fluoride toothpaste once a day too." Reminder: No matter what product you use, make sure you brush for a full 2 minutes.

The Quickie Guide to a Fantastic Smile

If you do nothing else, try one or all of these tips for a younger-looking smile.

1. Moisture, Moisture, Moisture Keeping lips hydrated with a rich balm containing SPF will soften, plump and protect. Your natural color will be more vibrant—and any little lines will be less visible, too.

2. Treat Skin at Night If you notice fine lines around your mouth or thinning lips, anti-aging ingredients like hyaluronic acid, peptides, retinols or phytoestrogens can boost collagen production, adding fullness and firmness over time.

3. Whiten Up Stained teeth are almost inevitable as the years go on. Luckily, those little whitening strips at the drugstore will brighten you up; give yourself at least three weeks to start seeing results.

4. Try a Primer Using a pre-makeup primer—or even your foundation— to smooth out the surface of your lips (and the skin around them) will conceal any deep creases and little lines. Plus your lipstick won't bleed, so your smile will look more natural.

5. Color...Use It! You want a lip shade that's age appropriate, but bright and youthful too (certain colors can even make teeth look whiter). Anything within the rose family is a safe bet, regardless of skin tone.

6. No More Matte A lipstick with a flat texture will highlight wrinkles. For everyday, switch to satin, liquid lipsticks or slightly glossy stains with moisturizing ingredients, like shea butter, vitamin E or glycerin.

7. Draw Outside the Lines Don't be afraid to use lip liner to make lips look slightly plumper. Tracing each side separately, from the corner of your mouth to the bow, tends to create a softer, more natural looking shape.

Smooth Your Skin 5

Your total-body approach to skin tone and texture: How to tackle dryness, visible veins, sunspots, wrinkles, and more.

"All women want the same thing—to look radiant and feel beautiful in their own skin." *– Iman*

Good skin doctors will take your hand in theirs the first time you visit their office. They're looking for signs of aging, which show up first in those delicate areas—like the back of your hand. "Women want to wear beautiful jewelry on their neck, tops that show off their décolletage, and they want to have nice manicures," says Paul Frank, MD, a cosmetic dermatologist in New York City. "Yet these areas are so commonly left out of their skincare routine."

It's not just your neck, chest and hands that change in tone and texture as you get older. Legs and stomach might have stretch marks and cellulite, your nails could break or become brittle, your underarms may jiggle, and skin may feel a drier and flakier. Like many of the issues in previous chapters, these problems stem from inevitable hormonal shifts, innate genetics and everyday damage—from sun, smoking, weight fluctuations and just plain *living*. "We can't go in swimming pools, or visit beaches, or take hot showers, and not pay a price," says New York City dermatologist Jeanette Graf, MD. "Total-body skincare is underrated."

Whatever's bothering you, the solution lies ahead—and rest assured that our panel of superstar skin experts can vouch for its success.

MINI-MAKEOVER #1
Soften Skin All Over

When you enter your late 30s or early 40s, you might start to notice that your skin has a new texture and feel, says Ellen Marmur, MD, a dermatologist in New York City—and more often than not, that's completely normal. "Your hormone levels are beginning to change, so you produce less oil," she says, "and the skin loses some of its suppleness." Then, as you make your way into menopause, those little lubrication glands dry up even more. What starts as allover dryness might become itchy irritation; what begins as a rough patch might turn flaky. Cell turnover slows too—meaning dead skin sticks around before shedding. "You need a ton of extra moisture to stay smooth and soft," she adds.

The thing is, moisturizing isn't just important because it can change the way your skin feels to the touch. It's also crucial because it restores something called your moisture barrier, which is "what will protect you from inflammatory skin conditions and environmental sensitivities as you get older," says Dr. Graf. She's talking about everything from acne and eczema to rashes and allergic reactions. The bottom line, then, is this: Well-hydrated skin will fight off redness, rashes, even wrinkles—staying younger-looking and healthier for longer.

Smooth and Hydrate

FIX IT FAST AND SO IT LASTS

First things first: Sun damage can definitely intensify dryness and irritation, so you need to apply sunscreen to all exposed skin daily—rain or shine, summer or winter (See: Your Guide to Allover Sunscreen, p. 167). From there, tackling that tough texture is all about exfoliation, and restoring moisture comes down to finding a lotion you love that you'll be happy to apply more than once a day. Here's how to do it right:

For skin that's just dry...

Exfoliate and moisturize separately. Dr. Frank recommends exfoliating one to two times a week. Use a moisturizing body scrub with a physical exfoliant (like microbeads or sugar) that manually removes dead skin cells when massaged into the skin during your shower. **TRY: Tree Hut Shea Sugar Scrub** ($17.94 for 54 oz; *7years younger.com/shop*). Your next step is to keep skin moisturized constantly. Apply a hydrating body lotion from neck to toe at least twice daily, making sure one of those times is immediately after your shower. (See: Habit Rehab: Rethink Your Shower Routine, p. 155.)

TRY: Your Best Everyday Body Lotions

Moisturizers are a matter of personal preference: Some women may not mind a heavy cream for all-day wear, while others need a formula that feels sheer and weightless. If you're not sure where to start, here are some suggestions:

- **Best for Morning:** You might want a lighter lotion gently infused with butters or oils, which won't leave much of a greasy or waxy residue on your skin. **TRY: Vaseline Spray & Go Moisturizer** ($5.94; 7yearsyounger.com/shop).

- **Best for Night:** Here's where you can apply thicker creams or body butters with heavy-duty concentrations of hydrating butters and oils– or ointments that contain intensive softening agents, like petrolatum. **TRY: Dove Cream Oil Intensive Body Lotion** ($7.99; at drugstores).

- **Best for Itchy Skin:** Simply tackling dryness with any moisturizer should help, but for extra relief, try a mild, fragrance-free lotion or cream that's labeled hypoallergenic. **TRY: Cetaphil Moisturizing Lotion** ($15; at drugstores).

Mix up an easy allover skin-smoother. As an alternative to drugstore body scrubs, make a paste of 3 parts baking soda to 1 part water, then massage it onto your body. "It's a great exfoliant and gentle enough to use daily," says Jamie Ahn, owner of New York's Townhouse Spa. (The best part: It's inexpensive too!) **Cost per recipe: 6¢**

For allover dryness with rough patches...

Try a multitasking moisturizer. New York City dermatologist Kenneth Mark, MD, recommends a hydrating lotion that also has alpha hydroxy acids, which are chemical exfoliants that dissolve dead skin cells. "Amlactin is my secret weapon that I recommend for all of my patients," he says. "It softens, smooths and hydrates all at once— it'll even get rid of the thick patches of scaly skin."

TRY: AmLactin Alpha-Hydroxy Therapy Moisturizing Body Lotion ($20.75 for 20 oz; *7yearsyounger. com/com*). But beware: Some concentrations of alpha hydroxy acids can cause itching, stinging or redness for sensitive skin, so start by applying once a day, post-shower. (See: Habit Rehab: Rethink Your Shower Routine, p. 155.) If your skin tolerates the ingredients, you can increase to twice a day. But either way, you'll probably want to supplement your routine with a gentler moisturizer that you can apply as needed. (See: Your Best Everyday Body Lotions, p. 152.)

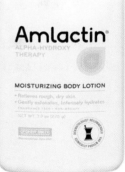

MINI-MAKEOVER #2
Erase Years From Your Neck and Chest

You may be diligent about taking care of your face, but it might be time to focus your attention a few inches south. Experts say your neck and décolletage can show early-warning signs of aging. "The skin there is much thinner, which means it may be the first place you'll notice things like sunspots and crepiness," says Ava Shamban, MD, an assistant clinical professor of dermatology at UCLA and the author of *Heal Your Skin*. Chalk it all up to sun damage—and not being quite as careful about your skincare routine in these delicate areas. "The first thing I always tell people is that 5 minutes of sun a day adds up over a lifetime, and this is perhaps most apparent on the chest," adds Joshua Zeichner, MD, a dermatologist in New York City. "I see lots of chronic damage in that V below the neck."

 ## Camouflage Crinkly Skin and Spots

You don't have to constantly cover up your décolletage with clothing! A few tricks can help you temporarily even out its tone and texture:

BONUS FASHION FIX
Get Rid of "Turkey Neck"

If loose, wrinkly skin around your neck and chin are bothering you, avoid the urge to "hide" them with mock neck or turtleneck tops or chunky jewelry, says *Woman's Day* Style Editor Donna Duarte-Ladd. Instead, draw attention down and away from the area. That means sporting more V-necks, scoop necks or button-down shirts (with one or two buttons unbuttoned), as well as one longer, more delicate necklace that hits mid-chest, between your neck and cleavage.

- **Moisturize.** Just like with any skin that's showing signs of wrinkling, keeping the neck and chest moist will make them look instantly tighter and smoother. And know this: Choosing a lotion or cream with hyaluronic acid will help hold that moisture in, for a temporarily plumper appearance. **TRY: CeraVe Moisturizing Cream** ($15; *7yearsyounger.com/shop*).

- **Smooth with makeup.** The makeup artists we talked to all agreed: You should be extending your foundation, BB cream or CC cream down onto your neck and up around your ears. And if your chest is also a problem area, go ahead and apply your base layer there as well. "I use a liquid foundation, pump it onto my

HABIT REHAB
Rethink Your Shower Routine

It may seem counterintuitive but frequent showers can zap moisture from skin. Here's how to overhaul the time you spend scrubbing so you'll achieve a healthier, more hydrated, smoother allover surface.

- **Turn down the temperature.** Hot showers may feel like they're soothing the dryness, but heat actually strips the natural oils from your skin. Water should stay lukewarm throughout.

- **Keep them short.** The longer you stand in the shower, the more moisture you'll lose from that critical barrier layer. "I tell people to play a song on their iPod that's less than five minutes," says Dr. Graf. "It's an easy way to time yourself."

- **Moisturize immediately.** Apply your moisturizing lotion within three minutes of stepping out of the shower, when skin is still damp. It'll seep into the outer layer, providing extra protection.

fingers, rub it together a bit, and then give the whole area one nice, sheer coat," says celebrity makeup artist Melanie Mills. If you happen to use a heavier foundation on your face, you don't need to invest in a lighter one—just mix a little in with your moisturizer, so it glides over this larger area more easily.

- **Target trouble spots.** You're probably not going to want to apply heavy primer, foundation or concealer all over your chest every day, but if there are one or two dark-and-blatant blemishes you want to hide for a special occasion, you can definitely cover them up with the same makeup magic you'd use to conceal spots on your face. (For makeup artist Laura Geller's easy how-to, See: Hide Spots the Right Way, p. 83.)

What Are Those White Spots on My Chest?

If little flat white spots are cropping up on your chest (or your back, arms or legs), don't be alarmed. It's probably a type of benevolent fungus called *tinea versicolr* that occurs in warm, humid weather and acts like a bleach that lightens skin, says Neal Schultz, MD, a clinical professor of dermatology at Mount Sinai School of medicine in New York City. "Because this infection lives only in the upper dead layers of skin, it can be treated simply with an exfoliating body wash that contains salicylic or glycolic acid," he says. Leave the product on the spotty areas for 5 to 10 minutes before rinsing. Repeat as needed to prevent more flare-ups. **TRY: Phisoderm Anti-Blemish Body Wash** ($4.69; *7yearsyounger.com/shop*).

Even Out Tone and Texture

For a longer-term solution, this three-step tweak to your skin-care routine will help to ensure that the skin below your chin matches the skin above it—which will shave years off your appearance.

STEP ONE: Protect it!

You knew this was coming, right? The key weapon in any anti-aging fight is sunscreen, so slather it on your neck and chest every single morning. "Prevention is really the best thing you can do, and it's never too late," says Dr. Frank. Use a sunscreen formulated for the face because it's gentle enough for this delicate area and sinks in quickly. (This rule applies even in winter, when your neck is the perfect target for UV rays bouncing off the snow.) **TRY: Clinique Sun Broad Spectrum SPF 30 Sunscreen Face Cream** ($21; at department stores) or **Yes to Cucumbers Natural Sunscreen SPF 30** ($4.24; *7yearsyounger.com/shop*). And if you're spending a long time in the sun? Keeping skin covered with the right clothing is yet another crucial line of defense. (See: Bonus Fashion Fix, p. 154.)

STEP TWO: Treat it!

"Make sure you moisturize your neck and chest every morning and night," Dr. Shamban says. "And treat these areas to the same anti-aging ingredients that are in your face moisturizer, like peptides to boost collagen and stop sagging and vitamin C to brighten and diminish spots." If you use a retinoid product on your face, you can apply it below the jawline too—but tread lightly, says Doris Day, MD, a clinical assistant professor of dermatology at New York University. "The skin on your neck and chest is less tolerant of very potent ingredients." She recommends testing the product on a small patch of your neck for a few days; if there's no irritation, start applying it once a week and slowly build up to more days. But if the skin on your neck and chest is too sensitive—or you're

7 YEARS YOUNGER MAKEOVER
The Problem: Damaged Skin

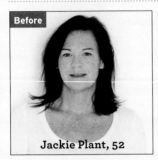

Before

Jackie Plant, 52

"I like being in my 50s," says Jackie, a food and nutrition consultant. One small matter of regret, however, is her time spent baking in the sun. Until her mid-40s, the self-described "beach fanatic" relied on a golden tan to help her feel younger. "I've done a lot of damage to my skin, and that's really what shows your age," she says. Even though she now wears SPF and a hat at her daughter's soccer tournaments, she wishes she "could peel off the sunspots—and start new."

THE FIX:

- **Wear Heavier Foundation:** First, the team from Laura Geller Makeup Studio applied foundation with a foundation brush to help provide even coverage. Then they used a concealer to cover and blend Jackie's darkest spots and blotches. (See: Hide Spots the Right Way, p. 83.)
- **Lighten Up:** Along with being diligent about wearing sunscreen with SPF 30 or higher, Jackie also uses a face cream containing retinol to help rejuvenate speckled skin and vitamin C to brighten her complexion. (See: Protect, Prevent and Lighten Up Dark Patches, p. 84.)

FINISHING TOUCHES

1. Protect Neck and Chest: Geller's team used the same products below Jackie's chin as they did on her face to make the whole area even-toned.

2. Brighten Eyes: They also applied a shimmery, pink shadow at the inner corner of Jackie's eyes to draw attention to her baby blues.

3. Put on Pink Lipstick: A glossy youth-boosting pink lip color instantly made Jackie's look pop and created a pretty focal point.

"
I'm on the
road to
healthier
skin!"
–Jackie

worried about burning through your pricey face stuff—experts are big advocates of neck-specific creams. "They're formulated to deliver anti-aging ingredients without irritating the fragile skin," says Dr. Day. **TRY: L'Oréal Paris Age Perfect Hydra-Nutrition Golden Balm Face/Neck/Chest** ($19.99; at drugstores).

STEP THREE: Exfoliate it!

Helping your skin shed its dead outer layer can do wonders to rid it of sunspots and any crepey texture, says Dr. Day. Plus, according to Dr. Shamban, exfoliation can *also* help the anti-aging ingredients in your cream penetrate better and work faster. So this means using a facial scrub on your neck and chest once a week, or doing a treatment with a chemical exfoliant, like glycolic acid. **TRY: Olay Regenerist Night Resurfacing Elixir** ($18; *7yearsyounger.com/shop*).

HABIT REHAB
Keep Yourself Covered

Obviously you don't have to overhaul your whole wardrobe to protect your chest and neck from the sun. But a couple of key pieces can help to save your skin. Here's what experts suggest:

- **Carry a scarf.** "It's a guarantee that you'll be safely covered," says Dr. Shamban. Choose dark or bright colors and a tightly woven fabric to block the sun's rays, and be sure to toss it around your neck while you're sitting outside or running errands.

- **Choose crew neck exercise tops.** "Too many exercise tanks expose the chest!" says Dr. Zeichner. So he recommends a higher neck and short sleeves in a moisture-wicking fabric. You'll still stay cool, but have added coverage in the spots where sun hits most directly.

MINI-MAKEOVER #3
Smooth Out Stretch Marks

Most often found on the stomach, thighs and breasts, these crinkly little depressions can crop up at any time in life when the skin stretches—usually because of weight fluctuations, growth spurts or pregnancy. "It's exactly what it sounds like," says Dr. Mark. "The skin has been stretched, and it doesn't spring all the way back to normal." As you get older, though, you are even more susceptible to these telltale red or white lines. That's because the little elastin fibers that give skin its bounce-back factor start to break down, thanks to genetics and damage from sun or smoking.

 Cover Them Up

Thank goodness these frustrating little lines are usually in spots covered up by your clothes! But if you happen to have marks that will be revealed by a tank top, swimsuit or pair of shorts, relax. You can conceal them easily, says Geller.

1 Keep a good waterproof body makeup on hand for those occasions, says Geller: "It's specifically designed to conceal these types of discolorations." **TRY: Dermablend Leg and Body Cover SPF 15** ($28; *7yearsyounger.com/shop*).

2 Put some on a sponge applicator, then apply it to the affected area. Feather it outward, to blend it into the surrounding skin.

3 If you're not going swimming, set it all by patting on a translucent powder, which will ensure the makeup won't transfer to clothes. **TRY: e.l.f. Studio High Definition Powder** ($5.99; *7yearsyounger.com/shop*).

One quick note to add: If you have an area (like the thighs or stomach) spotted by several bothersome blemishes or stretch marks, you might want to consider applying an allover self-tanner, bronzing lotion or leg makeup. (See: Give Legs a Glow, p. 171.)

Catch Them Early

Sadly, there's no miracle solution for old stretch marks (these are the ones that already appear white-ish in color), but fresh ones—which will have a reddish tinge—tend to respond better to treatments. The most effective approach would be to have a dermatologist resurface the area with a laser, but it's costly—anywhere from $1,000 to $4,000, depending on the size of the mark. Since that's not likely to be in your beauty budget, know that topical treatments can help new marks too. Your best bet is to try a face cream with retinol, which—when rubbed on the area nightly—"may help smooth stretch marks and fade their color somewhat," says dermatologist Diane Berson, MD. **TRY: Neutrogena Rapid Wrinkle Repair Serum** ($18.41; *7yearsyounger.com/ shop*). Dr. Mark says there's some evidence that products containing soy or lactic acid may also lessen the appearance of new stretch marks. **TRY: Philosophy Take a Deep Breath Oil-Free Energizing Oxygen Gel Cream Moisturizer** ($34; *7yearsyounger.com/ shop*). The bottom line, though, is this: Marks may fade, but don't expect any treatment to erase them completely.

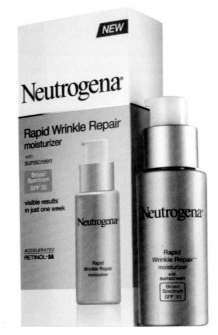

Make Your Hands Look Younger

Like the skin on the neck and chest, the skin on the back of your hands is extremely thin and delicate. Add the surprising amount of time they have spent soaking up sun over the years (just think about how often you're driving, with your hands propped up on the steering wheel!)—and you have a recipe for accelerated aging. "If you don't protect your hands well with sunscreen, you'll get that thinned-out, crepey, spotted look," says Dr. Mark. But you can keep them looking young and smooth by targeting two of the most common aging-related concerns.

MINI-MAKEOVER #4
Smooth Out Crepiness

What's causing this wrinkly, slack skin? As age dampens down oil production and erodes the skin's collagen fibers, your hands don't just get dry all over, the skin also becomes thinner, which could make veins more visible and wrinkles more apparent.

 Keep Hands Moist

As you probably already know from reading elsewhere in this book, well-hydrated skin instantly looks less wrinkly—but we'll repeat it one more time for good measure! When you add moisture, that moisture seeps in and plumps the skin, temporarily smoothing its surface. So give your hands repeated TLC. "Areas like the hands need more regular lubrication than the face, because the face has a lot more oil glands on it," says Dr. Frank. Moisturize morning and night, and toss a hydrating hand cream in your purse to re-up every time you wash your hands—which could cause extra drying.

Repair Skin Overnight

If thin, crepey skin on your hands is your biggest aging issue, you could consider using a collagen-stimulating anti-aging serum or cream, says Dr. Frank. But know this: It might not be your best use of money. "The further you go away from your heart—like the hands and the feet—the less the circulation, and the more difficult they are to treat," he says. "That even goes for in-office procedures, like lasers." Instead, Dr. Frank usually recommends this easy (and cheap!) at-home treatment for his patients: First, put on a heavier, petroleum jelly–based ointment before bed, then slip on a pair of cotton gloves or socks and go to sleep. "For women who complain about crinkly or dry skin, it really works wonders to restore suppleness," he says. **TRY: Aquaphor Healing Ointment** ($13.89 for 14 oz; *7yearsyounger.com/shop*).

TRY: The Best Hand Creams

The Good Housekeeping Institute lab-tested 22 moisturizing creams, then had 260 testers rate them on scent, silkiness and how the cream made their skin, nails and cuticles feel. These three—all of which kept hydrating six hours after application—came out on top.

- **Best Overall: Eucerin Intensive Repair** ($8.99 for 16.9 oz; *7yearsyounger.com/shop*) This scent-free, nongreasy purse-size potion creamed the competition on hydration.

- **Best Splurge: Aveda Hand Relief** ($21.95 for 4.2 oz; *7yearsyounger.com/shop*) Pick this citrusy star, loaded with plant extracts, for quick absorption, major moisture and nice conditioning for nails.

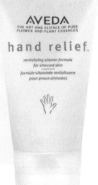

MINI-MAKEOVER #5
Fade Sunspots

These flat brown marks—which may also show up on your shoulders or arms—are hard evidence of years of UV exposure, say experts. (Oh, and despite what you've always been told, they've got nothing to do with your liver!) What happens is this: Sun damage sends pigment cells into overdrive, causing them to produce more and more of a brown pigment called melanin. "Age spots are usually not dangerous, but it's best to visit a dermatologist to have them monitored," says Elizabeth Tanzi, MD, dermatologist and codirector of the Washington Institute of Dermatologic Laser Surgery in Washington, DC. Skin cancer concerns aside, you'll probably also be pretty eager to fade these marks—so here's your best-laid plan for evening out your skin tone.

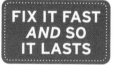

Protect, Prevent, Lighten Up

There are things you can do to minimize the appearance of spots, but first you have to protect them—and prevent new ones from popping up.

STEP ONE: Protect Skin.

By now, this should go without saying, but it's extra critical in the case of hyperpigmentation. No matter what you do to lighten up, say experts, spots will keep popping up—and existing ones will get darker again—if you don't shield those sun-damaged pigment cells from more UV exposure. Applying regular sunscreen of SPF 30 or more in the morning (and again every two hours in direct sun) should do the trick, but you could also invest in a good, purse-size, all-in-one SPF-infused hand moisturizer for extra protection and hydration. **TRY: Paula's Choice Resist Ultimate Anti-Aging Hand Cream SPF 30** ($13; *paulaschoice.com*).

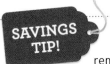

SAVINGS TIP!

Fade sunspots with lemon juice. This at-home remedy is an exfoliant *and* spot-fader in one:

- **The citric acid** helps dissolve dead skin cells, exposing fresh skin underneath

- **The vitamin C** is an antioxidant that protects the skin from future damage

HOW TO USE IT: Cut the fruit in half and squeeze out the juice. Dab on skin with a cotton swab and leave on for 1 to 2 minutes before rinsing. Use this remedy before bed, but not in the morning (citrus contains a compound that can cause darkening when exposed to sunlight). **Cost per recipe: 33¢**

(For more advice on treating sunspots on your face, See: Make Sun Damage Disappear, p. 83.)

STEP TWO: Fade Dark Spots.

To minimize the appearance of spots that already exist, try a twice-daily application of a serum or cream that's formulated with known lightening agents, like vitamin C or kojic acid. **TRY: Yes to Grapefruit Dark Spot Correcting Serum** ($16.69; *7yearsyounger.com/shop*) or **Clinique Even Better Clinical Dark Spot Corrector** ($39.70; *7yearsyounger.com/shop*). Exfoliation—which will slough off the top layer of dark, dead cells—can help too. "It's probably not going to take away all of the brown spots, but it can even you out," says Dr. Tanzi. So treat hands with a scrub or lotion with glycolic acid once a week. **TRY: Avon Anew Clinical Absolute Even Hand Cream SPF 15** ($8; *avon.com*).

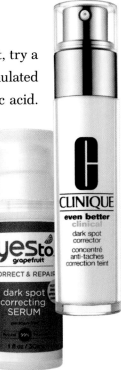

Your Guide to Allover Sunscreen

Ready to enjoy the great outdoors? Your skin needs extra protection—especially between 10 A.M. and 4 P.M., when the sun is strongest. "Even if you're under an umbrella or hat, UV rays can still reach you by reflecting off water, sand or rocks," says Dr. Shamban. And if you've considered skipping SPF, don't—a week off can undo a year's worth of protection! Target specific areas:

- **Lotions:** Slather on SPF 30 or higher on *every* area of skin—face, front and back torso, each arm, and each leg—at least 30 minutes before heading outdoors. **TRY: Neutrogena Beach Defense Sunscreen Lotion Broad Spectrum SPF 70** ($9.33; *7yearsyounger.com/shop*).

- **Sticks:** Spot-treat the places you always seem to forget: tops of ears, tip of nose, cheeks, even feet. **TRY: Yes to Cucumbers Soothing Natural Sunscreen SPF 30 Stick** ($8.97; *7yearsyounger.com/shop*).

- **Spray:** The rule is to reapply sunscreen every 2 hours or after taking a dip. A spray with SPF 30 or higher makes application easier—just spritz it and rub it in. **TRY: Hawaiian Tropic Silk Hydration Sunscreen Clear Mist Spray SPF 30** ($9.99; at drugstores).

More Sunscreen Tips

- **Load Up:** You need a *lot* of lotion to be properly protected. In fact, new guidelines say to use a teaspoon on each arm, each leg, and your face, head and neck. Then, use two on your front/back torso and each leg.

- **Mark the Date:** Once a sunscreen bottle is opened, it's good for two to three years, regardless of the expiration date listed, if it's stored in a dark, dry place in between seasons. (But keep in mind: If one bottle lasts you the entire summer, you're probably not using enough.)

- **Check the Label:** Don't just look at the SPF. If you're planning on swimming, sunscreens labeled "water-resistant" will protect you for up to 40 minutes, while those labeled "very water-resistant" will protect you for up to 80 minutes.

MINI-MAKEOVER #6
Firm and Flatter Your Arms

When it comes to your arms, you're probably most concerned with your underarm jiggle—where did it come from, and what, exactly, is making it worse as you get older? It's a bit complicated, but here's your short answer: Thanks to the fact that your skin is losing elasticity, it becomes especially vulnerable—not just to the weight of gravity, but also to the weight of fat. That's when it starts sinking and sagging toward the ground. "It's like over-stretching a rubber band," says Dr. Frank. "You can only pull it so many times before it stops going back." A pallid, pasty tone and skin problems that cause bumps can certainly add to self-consciousness about going sleeveless, but worry not: There are easy ways to fix flaws and reduce that jiggle.

FIX IT FAST **Steal These Red-Carpet Tricks**

If you're going sleeveless in a few hours—or even a few days—all of the exercises in the world probably won't cause your upper arms to tone up in time (although a few quick chair dips might increase blood flow to your muscles, causing them to look more defined—and simply making you feel stronger and more confident). Beyond that, though, you can fake it, more or less. These insider secrets will help give your upper arms a tighter, shapelier, smoother appearance—before you even have a chance to rethink that sleeveless shift dress or tank tunic.

- **Firm skin first.** "You can reduce arm jiggle by smoothing on a cellulite cream that contains caffeine, which tightens skin for a few hours," says Meghan O'Brien, MD, clinical instructor of dermatology at Weill Cornell Medical Center in New York City and consulting dermatologist for Physicians Formula. **TRY: Bliss FatGirlSlim** ($25.49; *7yearsyounger.com/shop*)

- **Create an optical illusion.** For nighttime and special occasions, a favorite celebrity trick is to rub dry oil (it seeps into your skin and isn't greasy) on your shoulders and biceps. "It makes skin look luminous and your muscles seem more toned," says Carol Shaw, makeup artist and founder of Lorac Cosmetics. **TRY: Fresh Rice Dry Oil** ($48; *sephora.com*). (It's pricey, but a little goes a long way.)

- **Even out flaws.** For a daytime fix, apply a bronze body tint to brighten up pasty skin and lessen the appearance of cellulite. "The color is subtler than self-tanner, plus it washes off," says Shaw. "But look for one that says 'transfer-resistant' on the label so it won't come off on your clothes." **TRY: St. Tropez One Night Only Lotion** ($9.99; *7yearsyounger.com/shop*).

Tone Muscles and Clear Up Skin

You can't get rid of excess skin without surgery, but a mix of strategic strength exercises and a few skincare fixes can firm up the wobble and smooth out the surface. Here's what you need to know:

- **To target the jiggle.** "While you constantly work your biceps and shoulders by picking things up—like those really heavy grocery bags—there aren't many daily activities that work our triceps, which is why we get wobbly arms," says Kristi Molinaro, group fitness instructor and creator of the 30/60/90 workout. But a couple of quick, strength-building exercises, like tricep dips—done a couple of times a week—can help to firm them back up. (See: Tighten Your Arms, p. 245.)

- **To soften flaky or ashy skin.** This is where you need a little skin-care regimen rehab, says Dr. O'Brien. Avoid scrubs, and use a soap-free body wash with warm (not hot) water. Then, apply a rich body lotion to damp skin to lock in moisture. Pick a formula with lactic acid to dissolve dead skin cells on the surface. **TRY: AmLactin Moisturizing Body Lotion** ($13.20; *7yearsyounger.com/shop*).

- **To banish bumps.** If you have small red or brown bumps on the backs of your arms, it could be *keratosis pilaris*, a condition that clogs hair follicles. To clear it up, exfoliate twice a week (See: Allover Skin Smoother, p. 153), and cleanse daily with a shower gel that contains salicylic acid," says Dr. O'Brien. **TRY: Neutrogena Body Clear Body Wash Pink Grapefruit** ($9.99; *7yearsyounger.com/shop*).

ASK THE EXPERTS
What Are These Tiny Growths in My Armpit?

If they look like small, soft pieces of hanging skin, they're likely skin tags—benign growths the size of a grain of rice that can form almost anywhere on your body, often due to the rubbing of skin against skin (the armpits and neck are common spots). "About half of women have at least one tag," says dermatologist Robert T. Anolik, MD. Your fix: Keep your skin moisturized by swiping on a lightweight lotion daily. And don't try cutting off a skin tag yourself, says Dr. Anolik. Leave the snipping to a dermatologist, who has the proper sterile tools to do the job. **TRY: Cetaphil Daily Facial Moisturizer with SPF 15** ($13.99; at drugstores).

Love Your Legs

From visible veins to cellulite to stretch marks, a whole host of frustrating problems that come with middle age can make us a little less likely to show off our legs. Luckily, there are some issue-specific solutions—from the quick way to hide lumpy skin to the best ways to keep spider veins from spreading. Here, your fixes for two key issues. (See: Smooth Out Stretch Marks, p. 161.)

MINI-MAKEOVER #7
Hide (and Prevent) Visible Veins

There are two types of veins you need to know about. First: **varicose veins**, which are raised blue, red or flesh-colored lines on your legs. These pop out when a valve in the vein weakens, causing blood to pool. You can thank genetics, says Dr. Frank: "These are the bumpy, bulging, sometimes painful veins you see as you get older." Second: **spider veins**— clusters of tiny, weblike red and blue veins near the skin's surface that can form due to aging, exposure to the sun, simple genetics or when estrogen levels are high (think: pregnancy). Depending on the amount of sun damage you have and whether or not you've been pregnant or are on birth control, these can turn up at any time, really, but one thing's for sure: As we get older, our epidermis thins out, so skin becomes more transparent—and thus, veins more apparent.

 Give Legs a Glow

The darker your skin tone, the less you'll notice lumps and bumps—like varicose veins, spider veins, stretch marks (See: Smooth Out

Stretch Marks, p. 161) *and* cellulite (See: Smooth Out Cellulite, p. 174.). So try one of these strategies to fake an even glow.

Use body makeup.

For special events (such as summer weddings), apply a bronzing body lotion, like **Sally Hansen Airbrush Legs Makeup** ($12; at drugstores), to dry skin. It'll even out skin and minimize spider veins, and your commitment lasts only until your next shower. If the color isn't a perfect match, go a shade darker (you can mix it with a plain body lotion to lighten as needed). Before you head out the door, press with a paper towel to absorb any excess—but not too hard, or you could leave behind texture marks, advises makeup artist Landy Dean.

TRY: Your Best Self Tanners

There are many different ways to get a glow, but most semipermanent bronzing products will fall into these three categories:

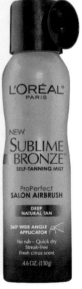

- **Gradual Bronzers:** These often include hydrating ingredients, and color deepens as you apply daily. **TRY: Jergens Natural Glow Foaming Daily Moisturize**r ($8.99; at drugstores).

- **Instant Tanners:** For your fastest fix, look for products that tint skin with just one application. They're different from body makeup because they don't wash off and typically last for up to four days. **TRY: Sephora Tinted Self-Tanning Body Mist** ($16 for 5 oz; *sephora.com*), **Comodynes Self-Tanning Towelettes for Face & Body** ($8.37; *7yearsyounger.com/shop*).

- **Airbrush-Style Sprays:** A wide, steady stream of color coats skin evenly, for streak-free results all over—including hard-to-reach areas. These are especially good for beginners. **TRY: L'Oréal Paris Sublime Bronze ProPerfect Salon Airbrush Mist** ($9.29; *7yearsyounger.com/shop*).

Get a flawless self-tan.

For longer-lasting color, makeup artists and dermatologists agree: Use self-tanner to give yourself a glow. Here's your step-by-step guide to applying.

1. Exfoliate. Use a scrub to slough off dead skin cells so tanner won't adhere to dry patches.

2. Moisturize. Put on your body lotion and let dry. To skip this step, opt for a moisturizer that's formulated to gradually tan skin.

3. Swipe or spray on. If it's a cream, apply the tanner as you would a moisturizer. If it's a spray, mist it slowly and evenly at arm's length—or according to the directions on the packaging (some will need to be rubbed in, others just set on their own).

4. Skip knees and ankles. Products travel up to an inch due to your skin's natural oils, so avoid these areas, which absorb and darken quickly.

5. Wash hands. A bronzed palm will give you away!

Change Your Habits

Unfortunately, once you have visible veins, there's not much you can do to erase them permanently—unless you're willing to shell out for expensive in-office treatments. (The methods differ for zapping varicose and spider veins, but both are pricey. And if you're prone to either issue, know this: The problem might pop back up in a few years.) All hope is not lost, however. A few simple changes to your everyday behavior can stop these veins from spreading—and keep your legs looking younger.

- **For Varicose Veins:** Put your feet up—whether you're sitting on the couch or at your desk. It will lessen the pressure on these veins and alleviate the often painful throbbing sensation that accompanies it. Also try eating a low-salt diet to lessen swelling, and avoid wearing high heels, which can prevent your calf muscles from pumping blood properly.

- **For Spider Veins:** You may not be able to stop spider veins from appearing, but you can prevent them from spreading. Wear support stockings if you need to sit or stand for long periods of time. This will increase blood flow and relieve the pressure on these delicate veins. The same goes for exercise—wearing spandex leggings will keep blood out of skin's superficial layer, so those tiny blood vessels won't break out, says Dr. Frank.

MINI-MAKEOVER #8
Smooth Out Cellulite

So you know what cellulite is—it's that lumpy, textured skin on your thighs (sometimes your buttocks or hips too) that resembles cottage cheese, or gives the skin a puckered, dimpled look. Maybe you've always had it (it's not necessarily age-related!), or maybe it has just now started to present itself every time you put your swimsuit on. Since it's caused by clumps of superficial fat being pushed out against the surface of the skin, your thinning epidermis (a by-product of age and damage) could be making it more obvious. "We believe it has something to do with the hormonal fluctuations in women, since most men don't get it," says Dr. Frank. "And a large part of it is also genetic."

One thing that's not to blame: your weight. Yes, despite what you might have been told, when it comes to your body size and shape, cellulite is an equal-opportunity issue. What will lead to its arrival, though, are weight *fluctuations*. So if you spent your 20s and 30s alternating periods of fad dieting with more lax eating and exercising habits, your yo-yo behavior could be showing its effects in your skin's now-lumpier texture.

Smooth and Firm

Despite what some cellulite creams might claim, no magic lotion will ever erase those lumps and bumps for good. But there are products that might help in the short term. "A cream that contains caffeine can make skin appear smoother for at least a few hours," says Dr. Shamban. How it works: The caffeine causes your blood vessels to constrict, which temporarily zaps fluid away from the surface of your skin for a short-term tightening effect. **TRY: Boots No7 Smooth & Improve Cellulite Treatment** ($19.97; *7yearsyounger.com/shop*). Then there's also the one tried-and-true, leg-smoothing standby: darkening your all-over tone with self-tanner or leg makeup (See: Give Legs a Glow, p. 171).

Build Lean Muscle Mass

"It's not what women want to hear, but the only real safeguards against cellulite are good habits and a healthy lifestyle," says Dr. Mark. The basics: Yo-yo dieting can make the skin looser, leading to more dimpling. Consequently, maintaining a healthy body weight—and building lean muscle mass in your lower body—might help prevent cellulite or lessen its appearance. How to do it? Incorporate walking hills or stair climbing into your cardio fitness routine, or perform other exercises that tone the glutes or legs. (See: Firm Your Backside, p. 246; Shape Your Legs, p. 247.)

QUICK TIP

Get the right fit. One of the biggest causes of skin problems on your feet: shoes that aren't the proper size. So always go shopping at the end of the day, when feet are at their widest, to help you find your best fit.

MINI-MAKEOVER #9
Give Your Feet TLC

Your feet have taken a real beating over the years. But it's not just that they've been bearing the weight of your entire body for quite some time, or have been crammed into pointy shoes—there's a bit of a biological explanation for it, too. Just like your hands, your feet are farthest from your heart—so circulation is poorest, says Dr. Frank. This means there's less blood pumping through them, and blood is what delivers everything your body needs to repair skin and fight off infections.

Probably the most common foot-related complaint is calluses. These patches of thick skin on your toes and soles occur when dry skin responds to friction or pressure by building up a tough, protective layer (you can think of it as your body's natural mechanism for preventing blisters). These calluses, when formed around the rim of the heel, can crack and split too—usually that happens when skin can't stretch under pressure from standing or ill-fitting shoes.

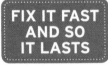

Soften and Smooth

Whether it's calluses, cracked heels, or just plain old dryness that's plaguing your feet, this easy at-home treatment plan should help:

DAILY: File and moisturize.

Do this every night before bed: When skin is still soft and wet from the shower, rub calluses with a pumice stone, which will smooth skin by sloughing off dead skin cells. Then, apply a specially formulated heel ointment or thick moisturizer that contains ingredients like urea (it increases the body's ability to hold in moisture) and alpha hydroxy acids (they're a powerful de-scaling agent). Slip on cotton socks and go to sleep—they'll lock in moisture, allowing your feet to hydrate and repair overnight. **TRY: Kerasal Exfoliating Moisturizer Foot Ointment** ($10; *7yearsyounger.com/shop*).

THREE TIMES A WEEK: Give them a soak.
One option is to do a DIY treatment made with the tropical fruit papaya, which has enzymes that help smooth and remove rough skin. Just mash up chunks of papaya in a large bowl, and rest your feet in the fruit for 30 minutes. Rinse and dry completely. You can also try a foot soak with urea, which softens calluses and scaly skin. **TRY: LCN Urea 15% Foot**

3 Pro Tips for Pretty Nails

Use these tricks of the trade to make your manicure last longer and keep your nails strong.

1. **Swipe on cuticle oil five minutes after your topcoat.** It makes the top layer slick and can help minimize nicks as your mani dries. (You should also apply it daily to keep nails flexible, which helps prevent chips and breaks)

2. **A good mani should last about a week, but applying a clear coat every two to three days post-polish can extend its longevity.** Use a clear nail strengthener rather than a fast-drying topcoat, which won't adhere well to polish that's already dry. **TRY: Sally Hansen Maximum Strength Top Coat** ($6; at drugstores).

3. **Keep polish on for 10 to 14 days, max.** (Once it starts to chip or peel it's stripping the nail with it.) And when you're ready to take your polish off, always use an acetone-free formula. Acetone dries nails out.

QUICK TIP

Pick the right color.
Still can't make up
your mind about
whether to go for Fire
Engine Red or the
Punchy Peach? Think
of the shade you're
considering as if it
were a piece of
clothing: Would you
wear a blouse that
color? If so, go for it!

Bath ($17.90; *7yearsyounger.com/shop*). Just be sure to follow up either treatment with your daily filing and moisturizer routine.

MINI-MAKEOVER #10
Get Stronger, Prettier Nails

There's a bit of a dilemma happening on your hands as you get older. Your nails are likely looking slightly sallow, or maybe the weakened edges fray. So you keep them covered up, giving them a weekly gloss or painting them with a new pretty color every time your polish starts to chip. At the same time, though, it's exactly this type of continual "care" that may be making them extra thin, brittle, stained or ridged. Paints and polish removers can strip nails of moisture and chemicals can stain them, says Dr. Graf.

So do you need to give up your nail polish? Not exactly. In fact, a good manicure or pedicure in a bold color can make hands and feet appear instantly younger. The key, though, is this, according to Dr. Graf: Giving nails a week-long rest from polish once in a while—and taking proper care to prep and hydrate them pre-painting. Your solutions lie ahead.

FIX IT FAST | **Do a Quick At-Home Mani or Pedi**

Painting your nails? It's actually the perfect way to distract from aging hands, says celebrity manicurist Deborah Lippmann. But when your nails are weak and brittle, you can't just throw on polish then scrub it off. You have to add a few strategic steps to the process—and know exactly how to file and coat. Here's our primer:

1 **Moisturize nails first.** Cover nails and skin surrounding them with a good cuticle cream first. **TRY: Sally Hansen Salon Manicure Cuticle Eraser + Balm** ($8.85; 7yearsyounger.com/shop).

2 **Pick a pretty shape.** The most flattering one mimics the arc of your cuticle bed. If it's round or oval, don't make your nails square or pointed. And file smoothly in one direction. Sawing back and forth shreds the multiple layers of protein and keratin that make up the nail, leading to peeling and breakage. (Note: For a pedi, you can simply clip!)

3 **Lay a good foundation.** A base coat doesn't just fill in ridges to make color go on more smoothly and last longer—it also helps prevent future staining. If your nails are weak, choose one that also doubles as a conditioning treatment (look for strengthening ingredients like gelatin and keratin protein). **TRY: Duri Rejuvacote** ($8.35; *7yearsyounger.com/shop*).

4 **Apply polish.** Put it on vertically up the nail to the free edge first, then paint horizontally right along the tip to seal color where it's most likely to chip. Add a second coat.

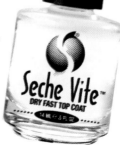

5 **Finish with a topcoat.** It seals in color and adds extra sheen. **TRY: Seche Vite Dry Fast Top Coat** ($8; Sally Beauty Supply Stores).

TO SMOOTH and SOFTEN...scrub, then soak. Aurora Dinu, a nail technician at Paul Labrecque Salon in New York City, recommends this weekly hydrating and exfoliating at-home treatment: Massage this sugar-honey scrub (1 tablespoon of each ingredient) all over your hands and nails for 1 to 2 minutes **(cost per recipe: 24¢)**. Rinse off completely, then soak for 10 minutes in warm, soapy water mixed with 1 tablespoon olive oil. Dry hands, then finish by massaging more olive oil into cuticles and nail beds. "Put gloves or socks over your hands and sleep with it on," she says.

Smooth, Strengthen and Whiten

Nails need lots of moisture, so hydrate them daily—every time you wash your hands, in fact. "A good cuticle cream or even an oil—like olive, jojoba or primrose—works fabulously," says Dr. Graf. And to work on longer-lasting repair, take a solid one-week break from polish every now and again. (Do it once a month to start, but as they start looking stronger and smoother, you can keep them polished a little longer.) With those simple changes, you're already on your way to healthier, younger-looking nails—but these targeted solutions will help as well:

- **TO STRENGTHEN...take biotin.** For thin or brittle nails, Dr. Graf recommends a good biotin supplement (also known as vitamin H), which "will increase the flexibility of the nail plate and enhance growth." Take up to 5,000 micrograms daily.

- **TO WHITEN...use hydrogen peroxide.** This natural compound can lighten and brighten yellow nails while you're on a polish break. To use it, mix 1 tablespoon 3 percent hydrogen peroxide with 2 tablespoons baking soda. Lightly buff nails first, then soak a cotton ball in the mixture and apply. Repeat daily until the yellow color goes away, which can sometimes take a week or more.

The Quickie Guide to Allover Smoothness

If you do nothing else, try one or all of these essential tips for more youthful skin all over.

1. **SPF Everywhere!** Use sunscreen with SPF 30 or higher any time it will be exposed—not just at the beach. (And don't forget the back of your hands—the skin is delicate and especially prone to sun damage.)

2. **Moisturize More** Hormonal shifts in your 40s and 50s cause drier skin, so always apply a lotion with hydrating butters or oils within three minutes of stepping out of the shower (it'll seep deeper into damp skin) and again before bed.

3. **Target Tough Spots** Using an exfoliating body scrub once or twice a week should be enough to keep skin supple and smooth. But if you still have rough or flaky patches? Treat those daily with a lotion that has skin sloughers, like alpha hydroxy acids.

4. **Go Below the Chin** The skin on the neck and chest is incredibly thin and extra susceptible to crepiness and sunspots. So extend foundation onto your neck—and treat your neck and chest with the same SPF or anti-agers as your face.

5. **Work It Out** The best way to prevent stretch marks, cellulite and wobbly underarms: doing regular exercise that builds lean muscle mass and keeps weight steady.

6. **Embrace Bronzers.** Stretch marks or visible veins? Giving legs or arms a glow with self-tanner make skin appear firmer and hide blemishes too. (These products have come a long way and can look natural.)

7. **Be Strategic with Anti-Agers** To cut costs, use an anti-aging lotion on your biggest area of concern (like your décolletage) and a regular lotion elsewhere.

Your Food Fix 6

Eat to lose weight, feel great and live longer—no dieting required

"What you eat is everything. What you eat is what you are." *– Diane von Furstenberg*

Maybe you've been bouncing around between diets for years, with varying degrees of success—or perhaps that magic formula of eating pretty well during the week (with some special splurges on the weekend) just isn't working anymore. Why, you wonder, do your jeans keep getting snugger? There's no doubt about it: Your metabolism slows down after age 35, at a rate of roughly 2 percent to 3 percent per decade. But whether this shift has you feeling defeated (who has time to cook healthy meals?) or inspired (bring on the diet!), you can definitely benefit from a different attitude. "Eating the right foods can catapult you to the top of your game by boosting energy, enhancing your overall appearance and reducing your risk for serious health conditions," says Joy Bauer, registered dietitian and author of *Food Cures*. "Sure, by simply cutting calories you'll lose weight. But by cutting calories while fueling your body with high-quality food picks, you'll slim down, plus look and feel years younger."

To be clear up front, however, this chapter isn't a diet plan—it's about making easy changes and simple swaps at every turn, so that each bite you take is crammed full of energizing, satisfying, youth-boosting nutrients that benefit you from the inside out. How did we do it, and what can you expect? The Mini-Makeovers in the pages ahead were designed with these three goals in mind:

- **Warding Off Weight Gain:** No strict calorie counting here— instead, you'll use these tiny tweaks to fill you up on less and rev your metabolism too.
- **Increasing Energy:** By upgrading some of your go-to meals and snacks, you'll get longer-lasting oomph every time you eat.
- **Making You 7 Years Younger:** Adding the key anti-aging nutrients we've identified will help fight off aging-related diseases, keep your brain sharp, make skin smoother, and more! (Don't worry—our suggestions are fairly effortless.)

And the best part? As these little changes and small substitutions become a seamless part of your life, you'll notice major payoffs in the way you look and feel. You'll have more confidence and energy, and with those youthful qualities (and your new knowledge!) behind you, you'll automatically make healthier choices—and crave the nutrient-dense foods that power your body best. It's a food philosophy we think you'll find refreshing, not to mention inspiring. "Making small, manageable tweaks to your diet provides you with a sense of accomplishment that fuels your motivation and takes you all the way to the finish line," says Bauer.

MEET YOUR FOOD FIX EXPERT

Joy Bauer, MS, RD, designed many of the recipes you'll find in the pages ahead. She is the nutrition and health expert for NBC's *TODAY* show, and a contributing editor at *Woman's Day*. For more nutrition tips and healthy recipes, visit *JoyBauer.com* and follow Joy on Facebook, Twitter (*@joybauer*) and Pinterest (JoyBauerHealth).

Build a Better Breakfast

First and foremost, you have to eat breakfast. Think of it as laying down a foundation for the day that keeps you steady and sane. These 7 Years Younger Mini-Makeovers give you just the right ratio of nutrients, so that you're set up to burn more calories and eat healthier all day long.

MINI-MAKEOVER #1
Do Cereal Better

There's no doubt about it: Pouring cereal out of the box, or heating up a quick packet of instant oatmeal, is one of the easiest morning meals. But if your breakfast is too carb-heavy, it's going to make you sluggish soon after—and set off sugar cravings later in the day. These tiny tweaks will balance out your meal, while also helping you pack in more age-defying nutrients:

1 **Check the stats.** Switch to a cereal that has no more than 150 calories or 8 grams of sugar, and at least 3 grams of fiber per serving. Also make sure the first ingredient is a whole grain: whole wheat, oats, etc. (For oatmeal, the easiest way to get it right: Skip the flavored instant packets and go with ½ cup plain rolled oats—they're typically cheaper, with fewer additives and zero sugar.)

2 **Amp up fruit.** Pay attention to the cereal's serving size, then toss in ½ cup of an anti-aging superstar fruit, like brain-boosting blueberries, skin-saving strawberries or potassium-rich bananas (they help manage blood pressure).

3 **Add protein or healthy fat.** Skim or soy milk adds protein, and you'll get bone-strengthening calcium too. But consider sprinkling on a few nuts or mixing in a spoonful of nut butter (for hot cereal), so that you get some heart-healthy fat as well.

Whole-Grain Cereal Crunch:

¾ cup bran flakes (such as Kellogg's or Post) + 1 Tablespoon pecans + ½ cup strawberries, sliced + 1 cup nonfat milk (or soy milk)

Peanut Butter-Banana Oatmeal:

½ cup dry oats (cooked) + 1 Tablespoon peanut butter + 1 small banana, sliced + sprinkle of cinnamon

Joy's Pumpkin-Chia Oatmeal Recipe

Oats are filled with a cholesterol-lowering fiber called *beta glucan* **as well as 4 grams total fiber** per half cup, which helps you stay full longer. This "beauty bowl" provides **beta carotene (from pumpkin) and omega-3s (from chia seeds)**, which nourish your skin for a radiant glow.

Makes: 1 serving **Cost per serving:** $1.36

½ cup rolled oats
½ cup pure pumpkin purée
2 teaspoons pure maple syrup
1 teaspoon chia seeds

½ teaspoon ground cinnamon
¼ teaspoon vanilla extract
1 Tablespoon chopped almonds

1. Combine the oats and 1 cup water in a microwave-safe bowl and cook according to package directions.

2. Add the pumpkin, maple syrup, chia seeds, cinnamon and vanilla. Mix thoroughly and microwave until hot, about 1 to 2 minutes (add an extra ¼ to ½ cup water if a thinner consistency is desired).

3. Sprinkle the nuts on top.

MINI-MAKEOVER #2
Do Eggs Better

Recent research has more or less disproved the theory that the cholesterol naturally found in food goes straight to your arteries. In fact, egg yolks are rich in omega-3 fatty acids, which aren't just good for your hair and skin—they may have protective benefits for your heart too. Experts say you can safely eat one whole egg a day, so here's our favorite way to work them into a healthy breakfast.

Joy's Super-quick Egg Sandwich Recipe

Microwaving eggs is incredibly easy. Just mist a mug with cooking spray, and add one raw egg (stirred). Nuke it for about 45 to 60 seconds, then pop the cooked eggs on a toasted whole-grain English muffin with one or more of these 7 Years Younger anti-aging boosters, full of disease-fighting, metabolism-stoking, skin-strengthening nutrients: $\frac{1}{8}$ avocado + 1 slice tomato + 1 to 2 dashes hot sauce

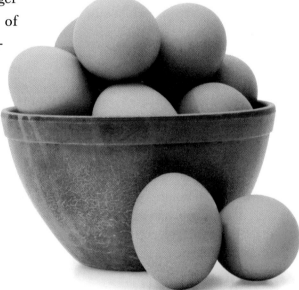

Joy's Fiesta Vegetable Omelet Recipe

Got 15 minutes? Whip up this antioxidant-packed breakfast. **Eggs** are a great source of B_6 and B_{12}—without enough of these nutrients, the hair cells can starve, causing shedding, slow growth or breakage. And diets with lots of colorful vegetables, like you'll find in this recipe, may help reduce menopausal symptoms, like hot flashes and night sweats. (See: Foods That Fight Hot Flashes, p. 211.)

Serves: 1 **Cost per serving:** $1.70

½ **cup onions, chopped**
½ **cup mushrooms, sliced**
½ **cup bell pepper, chopped**

1 **egg**
3 **egg whites**
2 **Tablespoons salsa**

1. Liberally coat a small skillet with oil spray and preheat the pan over medium heat. Sauté the onions, mushrooms and bell peppers until soft, 5 to 7 minutes.

2. In a small bowl beat the whole egg with the egg whites. Add the eggs to the skillet.

3. When the bottom of the omelet is cooked, gently flip and cook the other side. Fold one side over the other.

4. Top the omelet with the salsa and serve.

Grabbing Breakfast On the Go?

At a deli, drive-thru or coffee shop, your best bets will mimic the Mini-Makeovers here. Look for eggs on English muffins; unsweetened oatmeal with nuts and dried fruit; peanut butter toast (whole-wheat if possible) with a banana; and yogurt with real fruit (not fruit syrup). Skip fat- and sugar-bombs, like baked goods, biscuits and buttered bagels.

MINI-MAKEOVER #3
Do Yogurt Better

If you're already reaching for lowfat yogurt, good job—it contains a hefty dose of bone-boosting calcium, plus eating it every day has been linked to a lower risk of developing high blood pressure. But instead of simply eating a cup on the run or grabbing a parfait with a little fruit and granola, you can make it more filling—and pack it with 7 Years Younger anti-aging nutrients too. Here's how:

1 **Switch to nonfat Greek yogurt.** A 6-ounce serving has twice as much protein, which will keep you satisfied longer. Tip: Pick plain, which is significantly lower in sugar than the rest, then add a dash of vanilla extract or a drizzle of honey for flavor.

2 **Swap out granola for a fiber-rich cereal, nuts and/or seeds.** You'll still get a crunch, but this way, the cereal (use ½ the serving size) comes with less sugar (See: Do Cereal Better, p. 186), and a spoonful of nuts or seeds adds the hunger-taming trifecta of protein, fat and fiber.

3 **Add sweetness (and fiber) with a cup of fruit.** Berries are bursting with antioxidants, which help your mind stay sharp. (Researchers may have found a link between bright berries and reduced skin damage too.)

Berry Breakfast Parfait

6 ounces nonfat plain Greek yogurt + 1 cup berries + 1 Tablespoon chopped walnuts

Trail Mix Parfait

6 ounce nonfat plain Greek yogurt + ½ cup Cheerios + 1 Tablespoon pumpkin seeds + 1 Tablespoon dried blueberries

Joy's Quinoa with Yogurt, Grapes and Seeds Recipe

Quinoa, a hearty, protein-rich whole-grain that cooks in 20 minutes, is also packed with migraine-fighting **magnesium.** And **pumpkin seeds** are rich in **zinc**, a mineral that promotes a radiant complexion by helping skin renew and repair. Bonus: If you make quinoa and keep it in the fridge, this recipe only takes 5 minutes in the morning.

Makes: 1 serving **Cost per serving: $2.92**

1 cup quinoa, cooked
3 ounces fat-free Greek yogurt, plain (½ of a 6-ounce container)

1 Tablespoon roasted and unsalted pumpkin seeds
5 medium seedless grapes, chopped

Instructions: Spoon the yogurt over the quinoa and top with the pumpkin seeds and grapes.

QUICK TIP

Hit the freezer section. That way, you can keep eating berries (a 7 Years Younger anti-aging booster) come winter. Bonus: Frozen fruits are preserved at peak ripeness, which traps nutrients—and they usually taste better too.

YOUR FOOD FIX

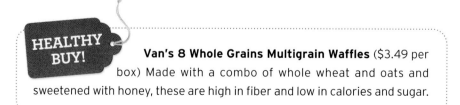

HEALTHY BUY! **Van's 8 Whole Grains Multigrain Waffles** ($3.49 per box) Made with a combo of whole wheat and oats and sweetened with honey, these are high in fiber and low in calories and sugar.

MINI-MAKEOVER #4
Do Smoothies Better

Your all-fruit smoothie doesn't work well as a stand-alone meal, especially in the morning, and here's why: Fruit is 100-percent carbohydrate, which makes your blood sugar spike, then drop—leaving you hungry (and tired) an hour or so later. For a breakfast that lasts, you need to combine all of that antioxidant-rich fruit with protein or healthy fat, both of which slow down digestion and prevent that sugar rush.

Tropical-Style Smoothie:

½ cup plain nonfat **Greek yogurt** + ½ cup calcium-fortified **orange juice** + 1 medium **banana** + 1 cup fresh or frozen **pineapple chunks** + ½ cup crushed **ice**

Chocolate Treat Smoothie:

½ cup plain nonfat **Greek yogurt** + 1 Tablespoon **peanut butter** + 1 frozen sliced **banana** + 1½ teaspoon unsweetened **cocoa powder**

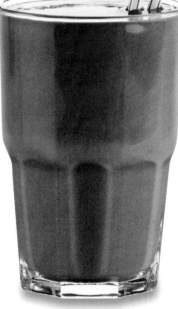

Joy's Banana Almond Energy Smoothie Recipe

Try adding **almond butter** to your smoothie, says Bauer. Almonds come packaged with **vitamin E**, which helps reduce wrinkles and blemishes by protecting your skin from sun damage.

Serves: 2 **Cost per serving: 73¢**

1 large banana, sliced and frozen	1 cup fat-free milk
2 Tablespoons natural almond butter	4 ice cubes
6 ounces nonfat yogurt	

Instructions: In a blender, combine all of the ingredients and purée until smooth.

MINI-MAKEOVER #5
Do Toast Better

You may rely on bread as a day-starting staple. But there are some pretty simple swaps you can make to both boost the nutrition *and* beat boredom:

- **Substitute rye or whole-wheat bread for white.** As a general rule, look for products that have at least 3 grams of fiber yet no more than 6 grams of sugar per serving. (Healthy whole-wheat frozen waffles work too, but pass on the bagel—it packs almost *twice* as many calories as two slices of bread.)

- **Skip butter or cream cheese.** Use something lower in saturated fat and higher in protein, with additional 7 Years Younger benefits, like natural nut butters, nonfat ricotta cheese or eggs.

- **Add at least one fruit or veggie.** The possibilities are endless—pears, apples, grapes, strawberries, tomatoes and avocados are nutrient-rich picks.

Nutty Pear Toast:

1 **whole-wheat waffle** + 2 Tablespoons **peanut** or **almond butter** + ½ sliced **pear**

Sweet Ricotta Toast:

1 **whole-wheat English muffin** + sweet ricotta spread (¼ cup nonfat **ricotta** mixed with 1 teaspoon **honey**) + ½ cup sliced **grapes** + 2 Tablespoons chopped **pecans**

Creamy Avocado Toast:

1 slice **whole-wheat bread** + ½ ripe **avocado** + squeeze of **lime juice** + pinch of **red pepper** or salt

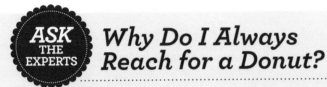

Why Do I Always Reach for a Donut?

It's not uncommon to crave carbs first thing in the morning, says Bauer. "Those cravings may be related to what you're accustomed to eating when you wake up," she says. "However, it can be connected to sleep deprivation or hormone fluctuations during your menstrual cycle or menopause too." But it's not the best way to fuel up first thing, says Bauer. The great news is, you can still have your "cake" and eat it, too. The key is finding a lower-fat, lower-sugar, dessert-inspired breakfast you love—one that *also* packs in protein. So mix 2 teaspoons unsweetened cocoa powder into a container of Greek yogurt before you build your **Anti-Aging Parfait** (See: p. 190), whip up the **Chocolate Treat Smoothie** (See: p. 192), or try the **Sweet Ricotta Toast** (See: *above*). And for help kicking a sugar addiction? (See: Beat Sugar Addiction, p. 227.)

Love Your Lunch

Whether you pack your midday meal or eat it at home, you probably choose it on autopilot by now (and there's a good chance it starts with S: sandwich, salad, soup). But there's only so much ham and cheese you can eat, and these healthy lunch ideas will break you out of a rut—while also adding the protein and antioxidants your brain and body need.

MINI-MAKEOVER #6
Do Sandwiches Better

It's amazing how many calories (and how much fat!) can live between two slices of bread. So why not choose fixings that are both good for you and delicious? This list will help you fulfill every opportunity to pack your sandwich full of youth-boosting nutrients while also keeping your waistline in check.

- **Start with the bread or wrap.** For the most nutritional benefit, make sure the first ingredient on the label starts with "100% whole." *Smart options: whole-grain, whole-wheat, rye, oats, multigrain.*

- **Pack in protein.** Anchor your sandwich with poultry, fish or another lean protein. Make sure deli meat doesn't contain nitrates (chemicals that may be linked to cancer). *Smart options: lean turkey or chicken breast, canned tuna or salmon, slices of tofu.*

- **Fill it with fruit.** This ups the fiber and nutrients and adds fresh flavor, sweetness and crunch. *Smart options: apple and pear slices, grape halves, raisins, dried cranberries.*

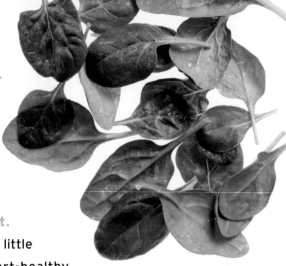

- **Layer on leafy greens.**
  They're packed with cancer-fighting antioxidants, fiber, and vitamin C. *Smart options: spinach, arugula, watercress.*

- **Use "good" fats—or no fat.**
  Instead of mayonnaise, try a little spread or add-on with heart-healthy omega-3s. (Or use condiments like mustards—just check that they don't contain high-fructose corn syrup.) *Smart options: avocado, hummus, peanut butter, pesto.*

Salmon Sandwich:

Drizzle 3.5 ounce canned **salmon** with 2 teaspoons **pesto**; place on 1 **whole-wheat deli flat** + 2 slices **tomato** + ¼ cup **arugula**. Serve with ¼ cup no-salt-added canned **chickpeas** + 1 cup **cherry tomatoes**

Curried Chickpea Pita:

Stuff a 6" **whole-wheat pita pocket** with ½ cup no-salt-added canned **chickpeas** + 1 Tablespoon **raisins** + ¼ cup grated **carrots** + 2 teaspoons **lime juice** + 1 teaspoon **olive oil** + ¼ teaspoon **curry powder**; top with ¼ cup nonfat **Greek yogurt**.

Turkey & Jalapeño Wrap:

Whole-wheat wrap + 2 slices low-sodium **turkey breast** + ¼ cup **black beans** + sliced **jalapeños** + **cilantro** + fresh **salsa**

Joy's Tuna Avocado Salad Recipe

Instead of mixing your tuna with mayo, mash it with **avocado.** This heart-healthy fruit is rich in **biotin,** a B vitamin essential for **hair growth and nail strength**.

Serves: 1 Cost per serving: $2.93

5 ounces light tuna packed in water, drained

2 Tablespoons diced avocado

2 Tablespoons diced red bell peppers

1 Tablespoon finely chopped red onions

1 teaspoon fresh cilantro, chopped

¼ cup fresh lime juice

Black pepper

Instructions: In a bowl, combine the tuna, avocado, red pepper, onion, cilantro and lime juice. Season with black pepper.

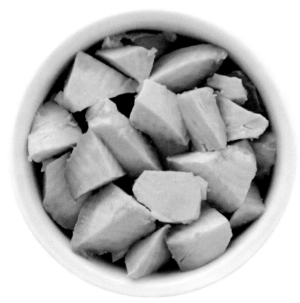

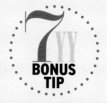

7 YEARS YOUNGER ANTI-AGING BOOSTER: CANNED SALMON

One 3.5-ounce can of wild salmon has 1,100 milligrams of brain- and heart-healthy omega-3 fats, and it also gives you 78 percent of your daily vitamin D, which helps to build bone.

YOUR FOOD FIX

MINI-MAKEOVER #7
Do Salads Better

These simple swaps will keep your lunch lean *and* pack it full of 7 Years Younger nutrients:

1 YOUR BASE:

SWAP OUT: Boring, nutrient-poor iceberg lettuce

SWAP IN: Leafy greens

Deep-colored lettuces will fill you up at less than 40 calories per 2 cups, and they are some of the most nutrient-dense foods on the planet. Load up on spinach, romaine or kale—they've got vitamins and minerals to preserve your bones, fight fatigue, and give you healthy hair, eyes and skin.

2 YOUR PROTEIN:

SWAP OUT: Breaded chicken, or no protein at all

SWAP IN: Grilled chicken, lean steak, low-sodium turkey breast, canned fish, beans, hard-boiled egg

You need lean protein at every meal (**TIP:** one serving of meat or poultry is about the size of a smartphone) to keep your metabolism humming and your hair healthy (See: Eat for Thicker, Stronger Hair, p. 38). Try a cup of black beans, white beans or chickpeas or a 3.5 ounce can of tuna or salmon.

3 YOUR DRESSING

SWAP OUT: Creamy fat-free dressings

SWAP IN: Vinaigrettes with healthy fats

A Purdue University study found that dressings need a little fat to help your body absorb the healthy compounds—like lutein and lycopene—found in vegetables, so go for an olive oil or canola oil-based vinaigrette. Add no more than a 2 Tablespoon serving.

4 YOUR CRUNCH

SWAP OUT: Croutons or bacon bits

SWAP IN: Nuts or seeds

Replace nutrient-void add-ons with almonds, walnuts or sunflower seeds, which add heart-healthy omega-3s—sprinkle on just 1 Tablespoon to keep calories in check.

Salmon-Strawberry Salad:

4 ounce boneless canned **salmon** + ½ cup sliced **strawberries** + ½ cup **grapes** (sliced) + 2 cups **spinach** + 2 Tablespoons **balsamic vinaigrette**

Healthy Chef's Salad:

2 cups torn **romaine lettuce** + 2 ounce sliced **turkey breast** + 1 **hard-boiled egg** + 5 **grape tomatoes** + ⅕ diced **avocado** + 2 slices **red onion**; toss with 1 tablespoon **olive oil** + 2 teaspoons **red wine vinegar**

Dijon Bean & Veggie Salad:

½ cup **kidney beans**, rinsed and drained + ½ cup **chickpeas** (rinsed) + ½ cup sliced **cucumbers** + ½ cup chopped **tomatoes** + ½ cup sliced **carrots**; toss with homemade Dijon vinaigrette (2 Tablespoons **cider vinegar** + 2 teaspoons **olive oil** + 1 teaspoon **Dijon mustard** + 1 finely chopped **garlic clove** + ¼ teaspoon ground **cumin** + ¼ teaspoon ground **black pepper**) and serve over 2 cups **leafy greens**

YOUR FOOD FIX

MINI-MAKEOVER #8
Do Soup Better

Broth-based soups packed with veggies and beans are generally low-calorie *and* lowfat, but beware: Cracking open a can for lunch (if you eat the whole thing) can give you as much as two-thirds of your recommended daily salt intake. To have your best bowl possible:

- **First: Go for low-sodium or "no salt added."** You should shoot for no more than 500 milligrams per serving. (Remember—that may mean just eating one serving, or a half a can.)

- **Then: Choose a lowfat broth or vegetable base.** Think: chicken noodle, tomato or vegetable over soups labeled creamy, chowder or bisque. This keeps fat and calories in check.

- **Finally: Amp up fiber.** Anything with fiber-filled chunky vegetables, beans, lentils, split peas, barley or wild rice will make it more filling.

BONUS: Upgrade It

Give a single serving of your favorite soup more staying power:

- **Chicken Noodle:** Stir in a cup or two of fiber-rich frozen veggies (like broccoli, spinach or kale).

- **Tomato Soup:** Blend in a plant protein like silken tofu or eat with a slice of whole-grain toast spread with 2 Table-spoons nonfat ricotta.

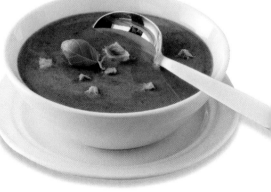

Joy's Butternut Squash Soup Recipe

Craving comfort food? Let the thick texture of **butternut squash** serve as a substitute for a heavy cream base. A single serving will give you a solid dose of **vitamin C and beta-carotene,** for more radiant skin. Cook it up on Sunday, so you can tote it to work in a Thermos all week. Paired with a small salad topped with chicken, beans or lentils, it's the perfect low-calorie, high-nutrition lunch!

Serves: 3 **Cost per serving: $2.02**

Oil spray
1 Tablespoon olive oil
2 large leeks, trimmed and chopped
⅛ teaspoon ground cinnamon
⅛ teaspoon ground nutmeg

1½ butternut squash, peeled and cubed (about 4 cups)
2 large carrots, peeled and grated
3 cups low-sodium chicken broth (may also use vegetable broth)
Kosher salt and pepper, to taste

1. Spray a large stockpot with nonstick oil spray. Add the oil and heat over medium-high heat. Add the leeks and sauté until tender, 6 to 7 minutes. Stir in the cinnamon and nutmeg, and cook for 1 minute. Add the squash, carrots and broth, and bring to a boil.

2. Reduce heat and simmer until the vegetables are tender, 20 to 25 minutes longer. Using an immersion blender (or a standard blender in batches), purée the soup. Season with salt and pepper and serve immediately.

MINI-MAKEOVER #9
Do Microwave Meals Better

Like soups, frozen meals are a sneaky source of sodium, too much of which can bloat you and lead to high blood pressure. Look for meals that have **no more than 600 grams of sodium and 4.5 grams of saturated fat**—bonus points for a short ingredients lists and whole grains too. Here's a 7 Years Younger–approved pick for every craving:

- **ITALIAN: Kashi Chicken Pasta Pomodoro ($4.49 per meal)** This cheesy pasta entrée has just 470 milligrams sodium (another good Kashi option: Chicken Fettucine Steam Meal).

- **MEXICAN: Amy's Light in Sodium Mexican Casserole Bowl ($4.99 per bowl)** This dish with a hint of spice is just 380 calories, with only 390 milligrams sodium.

HABIT REHAB
Drink more water

Your body often confuses thirst for hunger, so staying hydrated can help you prevent cravings and cut down on mindless snacking. And drinking more H_2O will improve everything from your skin to your digestion to your energy levels to your brainpower (a recent study found that mental reaction times are up to 14 percent faster after rehydrating with water!). For extra flavor, fill a pitcher with water and watermelon; frozen berries; mint; cucumber; or lemon, lime or orange slices.

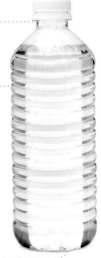

- **CHINESE: Healthy Choice Café Steamers Pineapple Chicken ($2.89 per meal)** It packs 18 grams of protein, thanks to the chicken and edamame (one of the best plant proteins there is!).

- **KOREAN: Saffron Road Bibimbop with Beef ($5.99 per meal)** It is stuffed with vegetables and contains only 35 milligrams of cholesterol.

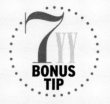

7 BONUS TIP

Tomato sauce is high in skin-saving lycopene. Add a side salad to fill you up, and give your slice a kick with crushed red pepper flakes.

MINI-MAKEOVER #10
Do Fast Food Better

When you can't avoid grabbing a slice or hitting the drive-thru, turn to these swaps, which will help you make healthier choices in a hurry:

PIZZA
SWAP OUT: Thick-Crust Pizza with Pepperoni
TRY: Thin-Crust Pizza with Veggies
CUT: 150 Calories

SUBWAY
INSTEAD OF : 6-Inch Tuna Sandwich
TRY: 6-Inch Roast Beef Sandwich
CUT: 190 Calories

WENDY'S
SWAP OUT: Spicy Chicken Caesar Salad
SWAP IN : Ultimate Chicken Grill Sandwich with Smoky Honey Mustard
CUT: 410 Calories

MCDONALD'S
INSTEAD OF: Grilled Chicken Club
TRY: Honey Mustard Snack Wrap with Grilled Chicken
CUT: 260 Calories

Make a Delicious Dinner

If you've been making healthy choices all day long, think of your dinner as a chance to finish strong. But on days when you've strayed, use it as an opportunity to get back on track by filling up on fewer, more nutrient-rich calories. These Mini-Makeovers are all designed to help you elevate the meals you already eat, so you can make small, seamless changes—for big results!

MINI-MAKEOVER #11
Do Pasta Better

Noodles often get a bad rap (thanks to the low-carb craze) but a plate of pasta is actually a golden opportunity to...

1 **Protect Your Heart and Stay Slim**
> **SWAP OUT: Plain pasta (made with white flour)**
> **SWAP IN: Whole-wheat pasta**

Eating three or more servings of whole grains (like whole-wheat pasta) a day can reduce your risk of heart disease, stroke and type 2 diabetes. Plus, whole grains are diet-friendly: One study found that women who ate more whole grains weighed less and had smaller waists than women who rarely ate them. Not ready to switch? Transition with a whole-wheat blend (like Ronzoni Healthy Harvest) or mix it (½ cup of whole-wheat pasta + ½ cup of regular noodles) until you get used to the taste.

2 **Save Your Skin**
> **SWAP OUT: Creamy Alfredo or vodka sauces**
> **SWAP IN: Low-salt marinara or meat sauce with ground turkey (at least 90 percent lean)**

Tomatoes are packed with vitamin C, which helps produce collagen, a protein that keeps skin firm, and lycopene, an antioxidant that protects your skin from the sun. (Your body absorbs lycopene better from cooked tomatoes, making marinara sauce a great source!) Jarred sauces can have tons of salt, so always choose "low-sodium" varieties—or consider using a can of chopped tomatoes with a little olive oil as a sauce alternative.

Tomato Zucchini Penne

½ cup grated **zucchini** sautéed in 1 teaspoon **olive oil** + ½ cup chopped canned **tomatoes** + 1 cup canned **chickpeas** (rinsed) + 2 ounce whole-wheat **penne** (cooked) + 1 pinch crushed **red pepper flakes** + 1 teaspoon dried **basil**.

QUICK TIP
Check your portion. Most people fill up their plate with too much pasta or overdo it when eating out. A healthy serving is no more than 1 cup cooked (roughly the size of a softball)—balance it out and bulk it up with a leafy green salad to start or a broccoli side, plus a couple of lean, protein-packed meatballs.

YOUR FOOD FIX

QUICK TIP

Sleep better.

Aim to finish eating dinner at least 3 hours before you hit the sack. Doing this will lower your risk of developing heartburn or gas, which makes falling asleep extra challenging. (For foods that help you snooze, See: Eat and Drink for Better Sleep, p. 278.)

Joy's Pasta with Pumpkin Meat Sauce Recipe

Pumpkin is loaded with nutrients (including **beta-carotene and potassium**) that will help your heart, bones, eyes and skin. Bonus: Potassium has anti-bloat properties to help you get that flat belly! Don't be scared to try this sneaky recipe—you can't even tell the pumpkin is there.

Serves: 4 **Cost per serving: $2.94**

1 pound pasta whole-wheat penne or rotini
1¼ pounds ground turkey (at least 90 percent lean)
26 ounces marinara sauce (Recommended: Ragu Light No Sugar Added)
½ cup pure pumpkin purée
1 cup shredded reduced-fat sharp Cheddar

1. Prepare the pasta according to package directions; drain, return to the pot and cover.

2. In a large skillet, brown ground turkey meat. When turkey is cooked through, add the marinara sauce and pumpkin, mixing to combine. Bring the mixture to a simmer.

3. Add turkey pumpkin-tomato sauce to pasta and toss. Fold the cheese into the pasta, mixing until just melted.

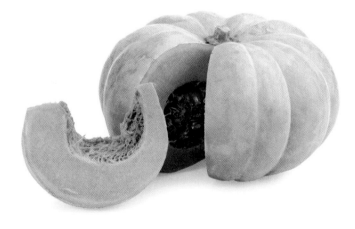

MINI-MAKEOVER #12
Do Tacos Better

Who doesn't love taco night? Here, three ways to make your recipes leaner—and boost their health benefits too.

1 **Traditional Ground Beef Tacos**

SWAP OUT: Ground beef + shredded iceberg lettuce

SWAP IN: 90 percent lean ground turkey + shredded romaine

The 7 Years Younger Benefit: Romaine still has crunch, but it's also high in energizing B vitamins. Switching from a fattier ground beef to the leaner turkey slashes saturated fat.

2 **Soft Chicken Tacos**

SWAP OUT: 8″ flour tortillas + sour cream

SWAP IN: 6″ corn tortilla + salsa with chopped avocado

The 7 Years Younger Benefit: Opting for the corn tortilla saves about 100 calories and delivers 100 percent whole grains. Salsa (with a diced avocado added) delivers skin-saving lycopene and heart-healthy fats.

3 **Fish Tacos**

SWAP OUT: Fried fish

SWAP IN: Grilled fish or canned salmon + shredded red cabbage

The 7 Years Younger Benefit: All colors of cabbage are a top source of bone-strengthening vitamin K, while salmon has a hefty dose of vitamin D, another nutrient that helps strengthen bones.

Salmon Tacos with Citrus Slaw

Two 6" **corn tortillas** + 6 ounce boneless canned **salmon** + 1/5 **avocado** (sliced) topped with 1 cup shredded **red cabbage** tossed with 2 teaspoons **orange juice** + 1 teaspoon **lime zest** + 1 teaspoon **rice vinegar** + 1 pinch **sugar** + 1 Tablespoon **chopped cilantro**.

MINI-MAKEOVER #13
Do Burgers Better

Burgers are an easy weeknight meal, especially if you premake your patties. Here are two easy ways to turn yours into a healthy dinner with 7 Years Younger anti-aging benefits:

1 **Swap Out Beef:** Lean ground sirloin is fine sometimes—it packs a potent dose of energizing iron—but switching to ground turkey (at least 90 percent lean) can slash saturated fat. Even better: Look for healthy recipes using canned salmon or beans. They're an even cheaper way to get plenty of lowfat protein and fiber.

White Bean Burgers

Sauté for 5 minutes: 1 **onion** + 1 **carrot** + 1 **celery stalk** (each chopped) in 2 Tablespoon **olive oil**. Stir in and cook for 1 minute: 1 clove **garlic** (finely chopped) + 1 Tablespoon fresh **thyme** + ¼ cup **fresh flat-leaf parsley** (chopped). Fold sautéed **vegetables** into: 2 15-ounce cans **white beans** (rinsed and mashed) + ½ teaspoon **salt** + ¼ teaspoon **pepper**. Form into six 1-inch-thick patties.

2 **Sneak in Some Veggies:** Bulk up your favorite burger recipe with finely diced vegetables. (It's a concept called volumetrics, and it allows you to eat more without worrying about extra calories.) Mushrooms work well because of their texture, but adding vitamin C–rich produce like spinach or red pepper to your beef burger can help your body better absorb the iron.

Joy's Spinach Taco Burgers Recipe

Spinach delivers a triple dose of wrinkle-fighting antioxidants: vitamin C, vitamin E and beta-carotene. It also contains two antioxidants (lutein and zeaxanthan) that may help to reduce your risk for macular degeneration and cataracts.

Serves: 6 **Cost per serving:** $1.54

1 ¼ pounds ground turkey (at least 90 percent lean)
10 ounce frozen chopped spinach, thawed and squeezed of excess moisture
1 packet taco seasoning mix, low-sodium

1. In a large bowl, combine the turkey, spinach and taco seasoning. Form the mixture into six patties.

2. Liberally coat a large skillet with oil spray over and heat medium-high heat (or preheat a grill pan or outdoor grill). Cook the burgers until they are no longer pink in the center, about 5 minutes per side.

3. Serve on whole-wheat buns with lettuce, sliced tomato and onion, and ketchup, mustard and/or salsa, if desired.

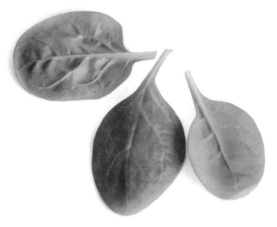

MINI-MAKEOVER #14
Do Stir-Fries Better

Stir-fries are fast, slim, cheap and can be loaded with a mix of disease-fighting vegetables. Plus, they make for a great leftover lunch—what's not to love? Here, two rules to make yours even healthier:

1 **Swap Out White Rice for Brown** You'll increase the filling fiber and get the youth-boosting benefits of eating more whole grains (See: Protect Your Heart and Stay Slim, p. 204).

2 **Replace Soy Sauce with Super-Power Spices** Soy sauce is high in sodium, which can cause bloating and high blood pressure, so use just a small splash of the low-sodium kind—then add flavor with:

- **Curry** Most recipes contain curcumin, a compound that helps control hormones linked to weight gain. Use 1 to 2 Tablespoons for the right amount of kick.

- **Ginger** It's a slight metabolism booster, plus its anti-inflammatory properties can help alleviate aches and pains from arthritis. Sprinkle on ½ to 1 teaspoon.

- **Turmeric** Thanks to its potent antioxidant dose, turmeric helps enhance immunity and improve digestion. (It might even help reduce your risk of Alzheimer's disease.) Add ½ teaspoon.

Stir-fry 4 ounce **pork tenderloin** (cut into strips) + 2 cups **broccoli, mushrooms** and **carrots** + ½ teaspoon finely chopped **garlic** + ½ teaspoon grated **ginger** in 2 teaspoons **peanut oil**; season with 2 teaspoons low-sodium **soy sauce** and top with 1 Tablespoon chopped **cashews**. Serve over ¼ cup cooked **brown rice**.

MINI-MAKEOVER #15
Do Potatoes Better

Ounce for ounce, sweet potatoes pack more vitamin A and beta-carotene than carrots *and* can help you peel off the pounds. A 4-ounce sweet potato contains 4 grams fiber, and because you digest it more slowly than a white potato, it's more filling. For an easy side to chicken, fish or lean steak, cook one in the microwave, then top it off:

- **Sweet & Savory:** 2 Tablespoons nonfat ricotta whisked with a drop of maple syrup and a pinch of cinnamon

- **Sweet & Spicy:** ¼ cup salsa + 1 Tablespoon lowfat shredded cheddar

Foods That Fight Hot Flashes

Sick of dealing with hot flashes and night sweats? The solution might be in your kitchen. A study found that eating a variety of certain fruits and vegetables can help reduce menopausal symptoms by 20 percent. For relief, fill up on these picks, which may help keep your estrogen levels in check:

- Garlic
- Peppers
- Mushrooms
- Strawberries
- Salad Greens

Joy's Baked Sweet Potato Fries Recipe

Make these **sweet potatoes** instead of deep-frying typical spuds to save tons of calories *and* fat, plus load up on **beta-carotene**. It's like nature's exfoliant, helping to sloth off old skin cells and lay down healthy new ones.

Serves: 1 **Cost per serving:** 80¢

1 sweet potato, cut into ¼-inch thick strips
oil spray
chili powder, curry powder or ground cinnamon
kosher salt and pepper

1. Coat a rimmed baking sheet with oil spray and spread the potato strips in a single layer.

2. Liberally mist the fries with oil spray and season with salt, pepper or any other favorite seasonings (ground cinnamon, curry powder and chili powder are all fun options!).

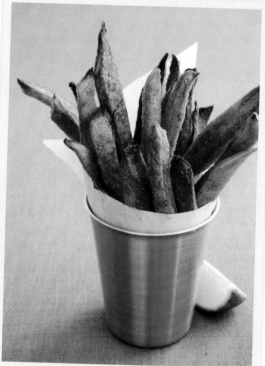

3. Bake at 400°F for 20 minutes, flipping the fries halfway through. Finish your fries under the broiler for 5 minutes to make them extra crispy!

Snack Smarter

Sometimes the advice about eating between meals is confusing. You've been told to snack more often to curb cravings, but "preventive eating"—when followed too closely—opens the door to overdoing it. If you're snacking between meals that are less than 4 hours apart, start by making over your breakfast, lunch or dinner *first*. (Adding more fiber and protein to your 8 A.M. breakfast, for example, should power you through to lunch.) Otherwise, use these snack makeovers—which target every craving—to find healthy bites to hold you over.

MINI-MAKEOVER #16
Do Fruits & Veggies Better

Yes, it's possible, and here's the rule: If you're not starving, then munching on some crunchy carrot sticks or grabbing an apple will likely do the job. But if you're feeling ravenous, adding at least a little protein and/or healthy fat to your fruits or vegetables will fill you up and give you longer-lasting energy. Your easiest options: 2 Tablespoons peanut butter; a handful of walnuts or almonds; ½ cup of skim or soy milk; ½ cup nonfat Greek yogurt; or ½ cup lowfat cottage cheese.

An Apple with PB Dip (Combine 2 Tablespoons natural **peanut butter** + 1 teaspoon **pure maple syrup** + a few dashes of **cinnamon**)

QUICK TIP

Make produce visible.
Keep apples and
oranges in a bowl on
your desk or kitchen
counter. Research
shows you're more
likely to eat them (as
opposed to going to
the vending machine
or raiding the candy in
the cabinet) if they're
in sight.

A Cup of Grapes with Lowfat Cottage Cheese (½ cup lowfat **cottage cheese**, sprinkled with **cinnamon**)

A Banana with Coffee + Milk (blend it as a smoothie: ½ cup brewed **coffee** + ½ cup nonfat or soy **milk** + 1 **banana** + 1 pinch **cinnamon** + ¼ cup **ice**)

Baby Carrots with Greek Yogurt Dip: ½ cup plain **Greek yogurt** + 1 Tablespoon fresh **lemon juice** + 2 Tablespoon chopped **dill** or mint

Yellow Pepper Strips with Black Bean Dip: 1 cup **pepper strips** + ¼ cup **dip** (See: Southwestern Black Bean Dip Recipe, *right*)

HABIT REHAB
Boost your food's benefits

1. **Stir-fry carrots or steam broccoli.** Chopping then heating them releases carotenoids, power antioxidants that may help fight cancer.

2. **Sauté leafy greens in a drizzle of olive oil.** The good fat helps your body absorb the nutrients that are released as the vegetable is heated.

3. **Let minced garlic sit for 15 minutes.** Exposing garlic to air once you chop it promotes an enzyme reaction that releases cancer-fighting compounds.

4. **Cut larger pieces or cook the vegetable whole.** Cooking bigger sections of vegetables like sweet potatoes or summer squash exposes less of the foods' surface to air and heat, which can destroy vitamins and nutrients.

5. **Boil potatoes whole. Keep the peels on, too.** This will help preserve their high levels of vitamin C.

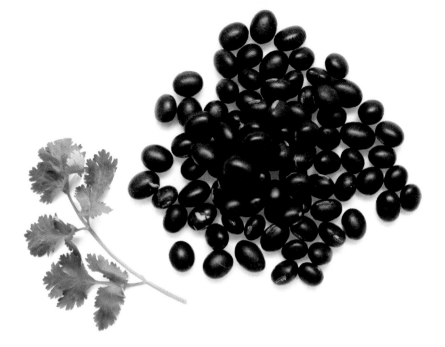

Joy's Southwestern Black Bean Dip Recipe

Black beans are rich in **zinc**, a mineral that helps hair grow strong and skin stay smooth and firm. Mix up this creamy, low-cal dip and keep it in the fridge—it'll make snacking on veggie sticks much more appealing. Just spoon out a ¼ cup first, so you aren't tempted to overdo it.

Serves: 8 **Cost per serving:** 47¢

6 scallions, chopped
2 teaspoons ground coriander
2 teaspoons ground cumin
2 15-ounce cans low-sodium black beans, rinsed

¼ cup fresh lime juice
½ cup nonfat sour cream
1 jalapeño, seeded and finely chopped
½ cup fresh cilantro, chopped

1. Coat a medium skillet with oil spray and heat over medium heat. Add the scallions, coriander and cumin and sauté for 2 minutes.

2. Add the beans and ⅓ cup water and simmer, uncovered, until all of the water evaporates, 5 to 8 minutes.

3. Add the bean mixture to the bowl of a food processor along with the lime juice, sour cream, jalapeño and cilantro and purée until smooth. Season with salt and pepper.

TRY: A Different Crunch

These crunchy snacks are made with nutrient-rich fruits and vegetables, healthy oils–and not much else.

- **Terra Exotic Harvest Sweet Onion Chips** ($5.89 for a 6-oz bag) One serving has just 40 milligrams of sodium per serving–almost unheard of in a chip or cracker. **Serving size:** About 16 chips

- **Barefruit All Natural Fuji Red Apple Chips** (99¢ to $1.49 for a .53-oz pack) There's one whole apple in each bag. The Granny Smith variety is deliciously tart and crunchy. **Serving size:** 1 bag

- **SeaSnax Classic Olive Grab & Go** ($1.39 for a .18-oz pack) These paper thin sheets of dried seaweed are roasted in olive oil and their savory flavor is surprising and satisfying. **Serving size:** 1 pack

MINI-MAKEOVER #17
Do Chips Better

These snacks will satisfy your craving for something salty or crunchy. Even healthier chips can be tough to put down, though, and the calories can add up—so be sure to pay attention to the serving sizes provided here.

1 Better Than Potato Chips....**Popchips Original ($1.29 for an 0.8-oz pack)** Satisfying those salty 3 P.M. cravings, these crispy bites have less fat, sodium and calories compared with regular potato chips. **Serving size:** 0 .8 ounce bag, or about 23 chips

2 Better Than Tortilla Chips...**Udi's Gluten Free Simply Sea Salt Ancient Grain Crisps ($3.99 for a 4.9-oz bag)** Crunchy and addictive, these grain-studded chips don't overdo it on the fat, calories or sodium. **Serving size:** About 18 chips

3 Better Than Nacho Cheese-y Chips...**Beanitos Nacho Cheese ($3.69 for 6-oz bag)** These natural white bean chips are lightly salted and packed with 6 grams filling fiber. **Serving size:** About 12 chips

Joy's Kale Chips Recipe

Kale is a leafy green busting with **brain-protecting antioxidants** that keep your memory sharp. And these healthy chips have just 35 calories per hearty serving, so they're a great snack to help you satisfy your snack attack.

Serves: 4 **Cost per serving:** 37¢

1 large bunch of kale
Oil spray
Kosher salt

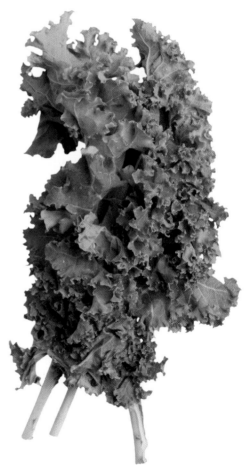

1. Heat the oven to 400°F. Coat two large baking sheets with oil spray. (The chips will be crispiest if baked directly on the baking sheet, without aluminum foil.)

2. Trim the stem ends off the kale and cut or tear the leaves into 2-inch pieces. Divide the kale pieces between the two baking sheets and spread them into a single, even layer.

3. Liberally mist the kale with oil spray and lightly sprinkle with salt. Bake until the kale is crispy to the touch and the edges are beginning to brown, 8 to 10 minutes.

MINI-MAKEOVER #18
Do Snack Bars Better

Many granola or energy bars hover close to candy bar territory, but these picks have the perfect formula for keeping you full (fiber plus protein, minus too much added sugar). Bonus: Their fat fats comes from healthy sources, like nuts and seeds. Look for a bar that's 200 calories or less and has at at least 3 grams of fiber.

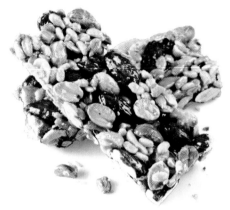

1 A Better Nut Bar...**KIND Nut Delight ($1.99 each)** Packed with almonds, peanuts, walnuts and Brazil nuts, plus nutritious flax-seed, these bars are sweet, savory and delightfully sticky.

2 A Better Fruit & Nut Bar...**Clif Kit's Organic Cashew Fruit and Nut Bar ($1.59 each)** Soft and chewy, this date-based bar is filling, with a hint of saltiness from the plentiful nuts.

3 A Better Granola Bar...**Kashi Chocolate Almond & Sea Salt Chewy Granola Bars ($3.99 for a 6-pack)** With omega-3 rich chia seeds, almonds and chunky chocolate chips, they taste like a treat yet only have 4 grams of fat.

HEALTHY BUY! **Sahale Snacks Grab & Go Classic Fruit + Nut Blend** ($1.79 for a 1.5-oz pack). It's packed full of cranberries, apples, almonds, cashews and pistachios, with just a touch of salt.

MINI-MAKEOVER #19
Do Trail Mix Better

Trail mix is salty, sweet and portable, plus you can pack all kinds of satiating super-foods (like nuts, seeds and dried fruit) into a single serving. The only problem? It's hard to stick to that tiny portion—and if you're not careful, you can easily eat up to 500 calories in a single sitting. So use this easy chart to make your own, which will fill you up for 250 calories or less.

1 Start with a Healthy Whole-Grain Filler **(50 Calories)** Add volume but not fat with: ½ cup Multi Grain Cheerios; 2 cups light popcorn; or ¼ cup Kashi GO LEAN Crunch Cereal

2 Toss in 1 Tablespoon Dried Fruit **(35 calories)** Choose antioxidant-rich cranberries, blueberries or raisins

3 Measure out 1 Tablespoon Nuts **(50 calories)** Pick dry roasted, raw or lightly salted almonds, walnuts, peanuts or pistachios

4 Add 1 Tablespoon Seeds **(50 calories)** Toss in sunflower seeds or pumpkin seeds

5 Sweeten it with ½ Tablespoon Dark Chocolate Chips **(35 calories)** For the most heart-healthy flavonoids, look for "70% cacao" (or higher) on the label

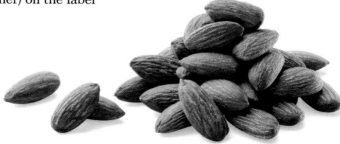

MINI-MAKEOVER #20
Do Dessert Better

These smart substitutes give you the flavors you love, but with less sugar *and* added nutrition:

1 If you love peanut butter cups... Try 1 teaspoon all-natural peanut butter on a square of dark chocolate. Eat it at room temperature, or pop it in the freezer and enjoy later as a chilled treat.

The 7 Years Younger Benefit: Peanut butter has vitamin E, a powerful antioxidant that's good for your skin, and magnesium, which helps strengthen your bones.

2 If you love apple Oie... Place 1 cup coarsely chopped Granny Smith apple and 2 teaspoons apricot all-fruit preserves in an 8-ounce teacup. Microwave at 50 percent power for 3 minutes, stirring every 30 seconds. Top with 2 Tablespoons lowfat granola and 1 Tablespoon nonfat vanilla Greek yogurt (150 calories)

The 7 Years Younger Benefit: Yogurt contains calcium, which can help relieve PMS symptoms and boost bone strength.

3 If you love ice cream... Purée 1 cup each lowfat **vanilla yogurt**, **berries** and 100 percent **fruit juice** (like pineapple or orange) and freeze into lowfat, portion-controlled pops. This makes 4 servings at 94 calories each.

The 7 Years Younger Benefit: Each pop has 15 percent of your daily calcium needs, plus the brain-boosting berries are good for your skin too.

Ciao Bella Blueberry Passion Sorbet Bars ($5.29 for 6 bars) Each pop is just 70 calories, making it a good alternative to a bowl of ice cream. Pair it with a graham cracker and it's still only 150 calories.

Joy's Cherry-Chocolate Ice Cream Sandwich Recipe

Cherries have potent antioxidants, called anthocyanins, which can slow age-related memory decline—so this sweet treat helps keep you young and sharp.

Makes: 1 Sandwich **Cost per Sandwich:** 64¢

¼ cup light vanilla ice cream (like Edy's Slow Churned)
6 cherries, frozen

1 full sheet chocolate graham crackers, broken in half

1. Soften the light vanilla ice cream and stir in the frozen cherries.

2. Scoop the ice cream between the chocolate graham cracker squares.

3. Freeze for 1 hour.

3 More Ways to Satisfy Your Sweets Cravings

Try pairing a dessert-flavored tea with something sweet and low-cal, like a frozen banana or grapes or a small portion of dark chocolate. Bauer's favorite combos:

1. Lipton Green Tea Passionfruit and Coconut ($2.49 for 20 tea bags). Pair it with 1 cup pineapple chunks (fresh or canned in 100% juice) or nonfat vanilla yogurt with 1 Tablespoon toasted coconut.

2. Bigelow Vanilla Caramel ($2.71 for 20 tea bags). Pair it with 1 square dark chocolate or 1 fun-size candy bar.

3. Celestial Seasonings Cinnamon Apple Spice ($2.49 for 20 tea bags). Pair it with a baked apple or 1 sliced apple sprinkled with cinnamon.

Targeted Diet Fixes

Easy solutions for weight-sabotaging habits or aging-related issues

MINI-MAKEOVER #21
Boost Your Energy

Food is your body's main source of energy fuel, but the wrong choices can leave you foggy, groggy and exhausted. Here's how to make smart diet changes that will give you more pep:

 The Energy Buster: Sugar Substitutes Since you can't digest them, low-calorie sugar alcohols—including mannito, sorbitol and xylitol—can cause stomach distress like bloating and gas, which are major energy drainers.

- **Limit sugar-free gum.** Not only does it often contain a sugar alcohol, but the act of chewing gum can cause you to swallow air—another cause of gas and bloating.

- **Cut down on diet or sugar-free beverages.** Instead, drink tea or water flavored with lemon, which will flush your system rather than make you gassy.

 The Energy Buster: Processed Foods That chocolate chip muffin or bag of chips will give you an express delivery jolt, but processed foods run through your system quickly, which means your energy spikes, then slumps fast.

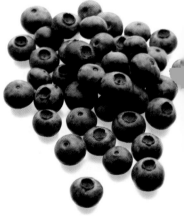

- **Less is more.** Eat whole foods as often as possible (fruits, vegetables, nuts, beans, legumes, whole grains)—and opt for the least processed versions of packaged foods, which have the shortest ingredients list. When it comes to pasta and bread, make sure the first ingredient is whole-wheat or unbleached flour. Foods that are closest to their natural state give you a much steadier, longer-lasting stream of energy.

- **Never eat sugar by itself.** Save the occasional candy bar, licorice or other sweet treat for after a meal that contains protein and fat, which will slow your body's absorption of sugar and prevent sharp ups and downs.

QUICK TIP
Ditch the energy drink. Most contain caffeine, sugar and not much else, so your boost will be short-lived. Instead, eat an energy bar with fruit and nuts (See: 218) or a handful of trail mix (See: 219), which has the perfect energizing combo of healthy fats, protein and carbs.

 The Energy Buster: Water Shortage When you're dehydrated, your blood volume decreases and less oxygen is delivered to your vital muscles and organs, which can make you feel worn down.

- **Drink an 8-ounce glass of water with every meal.** And enjoy strawberries, cantaloupe, honeydew, pineapple or, of course, watermelon at breakfast. These high-in-H$_2$O fruits will help ensure that you don't start the day at a deficit.

- **Pass on the nightcap.** Not only is alcohol dehydrating, it disrupts your sleep if you drink it within 3 to 4 hours before bed.

YOUR FOOD FIX

MINI-MAKEOVER #22
Rev Your Metabolism

Working these four factors into your diet is crucial

1 **Healthy fats:** Research has found that **eating fat for breakfast** turns on your fat-burning switch and helps your body use more calories all day long. Try these foods in the A.M.:

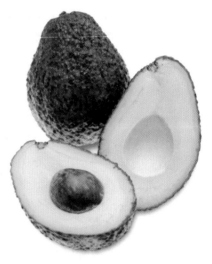

- 2 eggs cooked in 1 Tablespoon olive or canola oil

- 2 Tablespoons peanut butter on whole-wheat toast

- Sliced avocado on English muffin with 1 slice of cheese

2 **Cold water:** One study showed that drinking about **two 8-ounce glasses of chilled water** increased metabolism by 30 percent. So sip a glass of water (or unsweetened iced tea, which will also give you a shot of caffeine) with each meal. For added flavor—and vitamin C— drop sliced lemon into a pitcher of water and let it sit overnight in the fridge before drinking.

3 **Whole grains:** Research shows that your body uses more calories digesting **fresh foods,** like whole grains, versus the processed stuff. Transition to whole grains by following the "half" rule: In pasta dishes, start out by using half whole-grain and half white. Mix your regular cereal with ½ cup of the high fiber variety (at least 3 grams per serving).

4 **Spices:** Both **ginger** and **cinnamon** raise your body temperature, so your metabolism speeds up slightly to cool it down. Here's how to add it:

- Sprinkle 1 teaspoon grated ginger into oatmeal, smoothies and lemon-lime seltzer.

- Add a pinch of cinnamon to yogurt or a bowl of butternut squash soup.

MINI-MAKEOVER #23
Regulate Your Digestion

Battling constipation? It's common in middle age—thanks to a mix of stress, hormonal changes and a slower metabolism. Use these tips to keep your system running smoothly:

1 **Up your fiber.** Your goal is to take in 25 to 35 grams of fiber per day. To increase your intake, sprinkle wheat bran into oatmeal, yogurt and smoothies—you can even add it to meatballs and chicken cutlet breading—or eat more of these five fiber all-stars. It's best to spread them out, rather than bunch it up in one meal, which could actually worsen symptoms:

- Avocado (½ fruit) - 9 grams fiber

- Black beans (½ cup) - 8 grams fiber

- Blackberries (1 cup) - 8 grams fiber

- Dried figs (1 cup) - 8 grams fiber

- Green peas (1 cup) - 7 grams fiber

For example: Add blackberries to whole-grain cereal, have black bean soup for lunch and serve a side of green peas for dinner.

1   **Drink more water.** Fiber can't do its job without water—together they help move food through your intestines. Have at least an 8 ounce glass with every meal, and always keep a water bottle nearby, so you're sipping throughout the day.

2   **Take a deep breath before you eat.** It sets the stage for easier digestion. When we're tense, stress hormones spike, and these same hormones can disrupt the digestive process. To counter this, sit at the table and take four deep breaths, filling your belly and lungs with air, then fully exhaling each time. This automatically triggers your body to relax.

3   **Try coffee or tea.** The stimulant effect of caffeine can accelerate muscle contractions in your colon and bring on the urge to go. An especially good pick: chamomile tea. It helps relax the muscles around your GI tract. For the best relief, look for teas that are all chamomile rather than a blend.

MINI-MAKEOVER #24
Beat Sugar Addiction

Don't beat yourself up about your sweet tooth—many women experience sugar cravings and find it hard to stop once they start eating sugary foods, like cookies or candy. But it's worth it to overcome your dependency: Not only will it wreak havoc on your waistline, but too much sugar in your bloodstream can cause your skin's collagen to break down, leading to wrinkles. To reign it in, follow these three steps:

1 Cut out as much added sugar as you can. Do this for three days, avoiding both real and artificial sweeteners. Skip sugary packaged foods and drinks, including cookies, candy, cereals and soda—even diet—and stick with skim, 1 percent or soy milk in your coffee. Although artificial sweeteners are calorie-free, they keep the taste of sweetness on your tongue and can amp up cravings.

2 Add sugar back gradually. After three days, allow yourself one sweet treat each day that's 150 calories or less, like a cup of lowfat pudding or five Hershey's Kisses.

3 Choose foods that are individually wrapped. For example, go for an ice cream pop vs. a bowl of ice cream. That way, it's less tempting to go back for more.

MINI-MAKEOVER #25
Undo Diet Damage

So you overdid it this weekend. Don't be too hard on yourself—your metabolism speeds up when you eat a little more. To make sure a few off-track days don't turn into weeks of overdoing it, steer clear of high-sodium foods, drink plenty of water and get back on track:

1 **Take a 30-minute walk.** Do this first thing in the morning to jumpstart your metabolism and put you in a healthy-eating mindset for the rest of the day.

2 **Fill up on fiber.** Include at least one high-fiber food at each meal to satisfy you for fewer calories—aim for an extra 5 grams of fiber that day. Good sources include whole grains, fruits and vegetables.

3 **Make small cuts.** Trim about 200 calories from your diet, but don't skip meals. Eat a healthy breakfast, lunch, dinner and a snack if you need to keep hunger in check. And avoid any caloric indulgences like dessert and alcohol.

4 **Go for yogurt.** A few studies suggest that the "good" bacteria, or probiotics, in yogurt can help with digestion and may help ease bloating. Have plain lowfat yogurt to keep calories in check. To boost flavor, add a sprinkle of cinnamon or a small drizzle of honey.

The Quickie Guide to Eating Better

If you do nothing else, try one or all of these tips to eat your way younger.

1. Drink More Water. An 8-ounce glass with every meal—with plenty of sipping throughout the day—will keep your energy up, your digestive system regular, and your metabolism going strong.

2. Start Off Strong The right balance of protein and carbs at breakfast sets you up for success. You'll feel fuller, snack less and crave healthier foods all day long.

3. Make Every Calorie Count Pack each meal and snack with power foods, like leafy greens, bright berries, eggs, salmon and whole grains. These nutrient-dense calories will automatically keep your waistline slim, your brain sharp, your skin smooth and your heart healthy.

4. Shop Smart! Opt for the least processed versions of packaged foods, which have the shortest ingredients list. Foods that are closest to their natural state give you a much steadier, longer-lasting stream of energy.

5. Stop Before You Snack Don't munch mindlessly. Gauge your hunger before digging in—you might not always need something to hold you over between meals, but if you do, pausing first will help you make a healthier choice.

6. Pay Attention to Portions It's simple: Whether it's a packaged snack or a recipe, check the serving size—and stick to it. Even the healthiest foods will pack on pounds if you eat too much of them.

7. Spice it Up! Whenever possible, replace sugar (it's terrible for your skin) or salt (it's bad for your heart) with health-promoting, metabolism-boosting seasonings, like cinnamon, curry or ginger.

Your Fitness Fix **7**

Little ways to maximize your time and target trouble spots.

> ⁶⁶ When my body feels good, I feel more energized. I'm taking care of this body God gave me."

— *Queen Latifah*

I f someone offered you a groundbreaking, research-proven, doctor-approved youth serum—one that promised to safely stave off the signs of aging and make you feel younger immediately—would you take it? Well, that's what doctors and fitness experts say about exercise. Combining heart-pumping activity with strength-building moves doesn't just keep you slim, fight off disease and add years to your life—it adds life to your years. "In keeping your body strong and limber, you don't just look better—your self-esteem improves, and you feel like you can do anything," says physical therapist and fitness expert Maureen Hagan. To truly understand how exercise does this, let's break down the youth-boosting benefits:

- **You'll look younger:** You're already well aware that being active can help you maintain a healthy weight. But even while you're waiting for those stubborn pounds to come off, exercise is still working wonders for your appearance, says Ellen Marmur, MD, a dermatologist in New York City. "It improves your circulation, which gives you a natural glow and speeds up the skin's repair process," she explains. "And by shifting your fluid balance, it helps with bloating and puffiness too."

- **You'll feel younger:** Even a single bout of cardio can rid your system of life-zapping stress and replace it with mood-boosting brain chemicals. Once you establish a regular routine, though, that psychological shift and newfound energy will seep into *all* areas of your life. Research shows that you'll improve your overall health, your sleep, your sex life, your brain function—you can even dampen down the most frustrating symptoms of menopause, like hot flashes.

And here's the most motivating part: Whether you're already exercising or are just about to get started, there are easy ways to ensure you're maximizing your time, so you can cash in on every one of those payoffs. The mini-makeovers on the pages ahead are designed to help you effortlessly combine the two major types of exercise you need (cardiovascular fitness and strength training) to target your specific goals, while also incorporating other elements—like flexibility, balance and impact—that will keep your body and bones strong.

How to use this chapter

Ask experts how much exercise you really need, and you'll get a million different answers. But one thing they all agree on: You need to squeeze in as much activity as you can. So here's a baseline suggestion, but remember, it's important to be realistic. Start slowly, build gradually, and add more when you're ready—every little bit counts!

1 Do a cardio workout at least three times a week. Mini-Makeovers 1 to 5 help you maximize 20 minutes of your favorite aerobic exercises, like walking and doing the elliptical.

2 Incorporate strength training three times a week. Mini-Makeovers 6 to 13 target trouble spots or give you quick but effective ways to strengthen your whole body. You can do these mini-workouts after your cardio, or you can squeeze them in whenever you have 5 to 10 minutes. (Just be sure to give yourself a rest day in between, so your muscles can recover.)

3 Work on flexibility and balance two times a week. Mini-Makeovers 14 to 15 provide some of the stress-reducing effects of yoga while also keeping you nimble and injury-free. Balance routines can be done at any time, but stretching (which promotes flexibility) is best post-cardio, since your muscles are warm and pliable.

4 Change your mindset every day. After reading Mini-Makeovers 16 to 18, you'll see how easy it is to want to squeeze more activity into your typical routine—so that fitness becomes an effortless part of your life.

One more note before you get started: At the end of the chapter (see page 255), you'll find an exercise library, which includes a variety of flexibility and strength-training exercises with clear instructions and easy-to-follow photographs. Many of the tips and mini-makeovers will refer to these moves.

Fitness Fix: Revamp Your Cardio

How to boost the benefits of a 20-minute workout: Cardiovascular exercise (also known as aerobic activity) "is non-negotiable in your 30s and beyond," says Hagan. It improves cholesterol levels, lowers heart disease risk, increases stamina and blasts belly fat. Anything that gets your heart rate up to 60 percent to 80 percent of its max—where you're breathless and sweating—counts as cardio, but the trick is the more strategic you are about challenging your body, the less time you need to spend working out. Mix and match these workouts, which are designed to take full advantage of 20 minutes, three times a week.

Your Walking Workout

Walking is one of the best aerobic activities—whether you're just starting out or already exercising regularly. "Walking has more payback— physically, emotionally, intellectually—because it is a no-excuses workout," says Leslie Sansone, fitness expert and founder of the *Walk at Home* DVD Series. "When walking is your foundation, you're fit for a lifetime."

Here's the question, though: Is your daily walk—whether you're squeezing it in throughout the day or pounding it out in one swoop— doing all it can to keep you strong and healthy? Probably not—but you don't necessarily need to walk *more*. You just need to walk smarter! First, to get the weight-loss and heart-health benefits you need, your walk has to be brisk (For advice on gauging your pace, See: Ask the Experts, p. 240). But beyond that, there are a few simple changes you can make (like adding climbs or switching up your speed) that will challenge your body in new ways. So read on for three 20-minute walking workouts that will burn more calories and tone new muscles.

MINI-MAKEOVER #1
Walk at Home

Yes, you read that right. You can take a walk without leaving your house, and the workout below will be a lifesaver on rainy days. But don't just use it then, says Sansone—try to do it at least once a week. Why? "With traditional walking, you're using the same muscles again and again," she explains. "This sequence, by making you side step, kick and walk in reverse, fires up different muscles to tone you all over and keep you quick on your feet." Kicks and lifts also help you stay stable, since you need to temporarily balance on one foot.

You'll start with just the lower body:

- 2 min: Walk/march in place.
- 2 min: Do side steps: Step your right foot out to the side and bring your left foot to meet it. Then, step your left foot to the left side, and bring your right foot to meet it. Keep repeating until time is up.
- 2 min: Do kicks: Raise your right leg with knee bent, then kick it forward. Switch legs and repeat. Keep alternating.
- 2 min: Do knee lifts: Raise your right knee to your waist, then switch sides.
- 1 min: Travel: Walk forward four fast steps, then back up four fast steps.

- 1 min: Do double side steps: Step out to the right two steps, then step to the left two steps.

Now add the upper body to the same sequence you just did:

- 1 min: Walk in place and raise arms to the ceiling. Once they're there, hold arms above head with palms facing forward.
- 1 min: Do side steps, opening and closing your arms wide to the side with each step (palms should be facing forward).
- 1 min: Do kicks again, but this time, reach your opposite arm toward the kicking foot.
- 1 min: Do knee lifts, but add arms by touching your hand to the opposite knee when the knee is up.
- 1 min: Travel again, but this time pump your arms in front of you and back along your sides, as if you were rowing.
- 1 min: Do double side steps, reaching arms out to the sides and closing them with each step.
- 4 min: Walk around the living room (or up and down a hallway!) as you breathe deeply and cool down.

TO BOOST THE BURN Once the workout starts to feel easier, add 1 to 2 pound weights (no higher, to prevent injury) to build more lean muscle mass, says Sansone. Just set them down before you start the cooldown portion of the workout.

QUICK TIP
Cross-body movements matter. Any time you do an exercise where your legs or arms cross the midline of your body (like touching your right hand to your left leg), you're helping to keep your brain sharp, says Hagan. How? Communication between your left and right brains slows as you get older, but these movements force them to talk to each other, thus strengthening the connection.

MINI-MAKEOVER #2
Upgrade Your Outdoor Workout

This 20-minute routine was designed by Jessica Smith, a certified personal trainer and creator of the *Walking for Weight Loss, Wellness & Energy* DVD. It combines walking at different paces and resistance moves to burn fat, improve mood and strengthen your heart.

- 3 min: Warmup: Walk at an easy pace.
- 3 min: Brisk walk: Increase your pace slightly and drive your arms back and forth.
- 2 min: Squats: Do as many as you can. (See: Exercise #23–Squat with Chest Press, p. 266).
- 3 min: Power walk: Walk at a faster pace than your brisk walk. It should be difficult to maintain a conversation.
- 2 min: Box steps: Stand with feet hip-width apart, elbows bent and hands in fists. Imagine there is a box outlined on the floor in front of you. Step right foot to the top right corner, then step left foot to the top left corner. Quickly step back to the corners behind you (leading with right foot). Repeat for 1 minute, then switch and lead with your left leg.
- 3 min: Brisk walk: Talking should be tough but not impossible.
- 2 min: Side steps: Stand with feet together and knees bent. Take a wide step out to the right, tapping left foot into the right, then step out to the left, tapping right foot into left. Repeat.
- 1 min: Rope skip: Pretend you're jumping rope with an imaginary jump rope. Stand with feet together, arms at sides. Imagine you're holding a jump rope, and jump in place on balls of feet, making twirling motion with hands.
- 1 min: Cool down: Walk at an easy pace.

MINI-MAKEOVER #3
Beat Treadmill Boredom

This plan—created by Amy Dixon, star of the *Motion Traxx: Treadmill Coach* audio workout—uses incline and speed changes to help you maximize your machine time. Swing your arms as you walk to burn more calories and trim your upper body too.

- 2 min: Set a 2 percent incline and a speed of 2.5 to 3.0 mph
- 4 min: Set a 3 percent incline. Increase speed to 3.0 to 3.5 mph
- 2 min: Set a 4 percent incline. Increase speed to 3.5 to 4.0 mph
- 2 min: Set a 6 percent incline. Stay at a speed of 3.5 to 4.0 mph
- 2 min: Set a 2 percent incline. Decrease speed to 3.0 to 3.5 mph
- 2 min: Set a 4 percent incline. Increase speed to 3.0 to 4.0 mph
- 2 min: Set a 6 percent incline. Decrease speed to 3.5 to 4.0 mph
- 2 min: Set an 8 percent incline. Keep speed at 3.5 to 4.0 mph
- 2 min: Set a 0 percent incline. Decrease speed to 2.5 to 3.0 mph

TO BOOST THE BURN When you feel like you're getting fitter, increase your starting pace or incline and adjust the workout from there, says Dixon (increase incline at 1 percent increments and speed at .5 mph increments). Making sure your body is challenged (be honest with yourself!) will help you see continued results. You can also repeat the workout—or even the last 10 minutes—if you have extra time that day.

Three More Ways to Step It Up

Already have a walking workout you love? Sansone offers these tips to help you increase the burn.

1. **Tuck your tummy.** Pull your belly button back to your spine—this positions your body to reap the most benefits as you walk. "You're engaging more muscles, so you'll burn more calories and walk faster and stronger," she says.

2. **Shake it up.** When walking starts to feel easy, add intervals with a gentle jog. For example: Walk from one mailbox to the next in your neighborhood, then jog to the next. Keep repeating this walk-jog interval along your route.

3. **Climb.** This is the biggest booster, so add a hilly street into your route, or find a set of steps that you can climb a few times. "Even climbing up and down the curb for a few minutes will activate more muscles," she says.

Am I Walking Hard and Fast Enough?

To truly boost your health, any old stroll won't do. Your walk (or cardio workout in general) needs to be somewhat challenging. But what does that even mean? Experts say there are a few easy ways to set your pace—and gauge it during your workout—without relying on a heart rate monitor:

- **To establish your speed:** Use the bus stop test: Imagine you're turning the corner, and you see the bus has pulled in to the stop. "When you start hurrying up to catch it, that's the brisk aerobic pace that's going to bring you the best benefits," says Sansone.

- **To keep your pace:** If you walk alone, put together a playlist of upbeat songs (ask yourself: *Can I dance to this?*) and use the beat of the music to guide you. When walking with a friend, a brisk pace will make conversation tough, but not impossible.

MINI-MAKEOVER #4
Your Exercise Bike Workout

Just like switching up the speed and incline on your walk can help to boost your burn, adding intervals to a stationary bike workout will torch calories and improve your heart health. Try this 20-minute routine from Todd Galati, cycling expert and American Council on Exercise certified personal trainer.

QUICK TIP
Stand up to boost bone health. By standing up to pedal for short periods of time, you turn cycling into a weight-bearing exercise, which helps to strengthen bones and prevent osteoporosis.

- 5 min: Warmup: Pedal at a moderate intensity, about 70 to 100 rpm. (The effort should feel similar to steady walking.)
- 1 min: Tempo: Increase bike resistance and pedal harder. (Talking is possible but a little challenging.)
- 3 min: Recovery: Decrease resistance and pedal at a moderate intensity.
- 1 min: Climb: Increase bike resistance; stand up so that your bottom is off the seat. Continue to pedal from a standing position.
- 4 min: Recovery: Sit down, decrease resistance and return to pedaling at a moderate intensity.
- 1 min: Tempo: Increase bike resistance so you have to pedal harder.
- 5 min: Cooldown: Decrease resistance and pedal at a moderate rate.

MINI-MAKEOVER #5
Your Elliptical Workout

The elliptical can be a great cardio option—it's easy on the joints *and* it engages whole body. But instead of letting the momentum of the machine do the work for you, use this research-proven routine from Jessica Matthews, MS, an exercise physiologist and spokesperson for the American Council on Exercise, which follows the 10-20-30 training concept to maximize your time at the gym. It combines intervals of different intensities to burn more fat and blast away stress.

TO START: Set your crossramp (it creates an incline) to 11 and your resistance (it makes each pedal stroke more difficult) to 4. Because each elliptical machine is different, you may need to adjust. "If you find yourself bouncing as you pedal, apply additional resistance," says Matthews.

 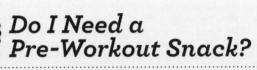

ASK THE EXPERTS *Do I Need a Pre-Workout Snack?*

If you're doing a 30- to 45-minute combination of walking and strength training within two hours of a well-balanced meal, you probably won't need more to eat, says Kristin Kirkpatrick, RD, a wellness manager at the Cleveland Clinic Wellness Institute. But if your workout is lengthier, or if it's been more than 2 hours since you last ate, eat a roughly 150-calorie snack containing about 6 grams of protein and 35 grams of carbohydrate 1 hour pre-workout (good options: an egg on a slice of whole-wheat toast, a cup of nonfat yogurt with a piece of fruit or a Luna Bar). This will give your muscles enough energy to work out for longer—and feel good while doing it.

THE WARMUP: Do **5 minutes** of pedaling at a jogging pace, which is low intensity to moderate intensity (this should feel like a 5 or 6 on a scale of 1 to 10, where talking is only slightly difficult).

THE WORKOUT: Repeat the following combination of intervals 12 times:
- **30 sec:** Start with your jogging pace (as described above)
- **20 sec:** Increase to a running pace, which is moderate to vigorous intensity (about a 7 or 8 on a scale of 1 to 10, where talking is difficult)
- **10 sec:** Pick it up to a sprint, which is vigorous intensity to maximum effort (about a 9 or 10 on a scale of 1 to 10, which is an all-out exertion)

THE COOLDOWN: Pedal at low intensity again for **3 minutes**, to bring your heart rate back down.

 TO BOOST THE BURN As you get more comfortable with this workout, capitalize on every minute spent on the elliptical machine:
- **Increase the crossramp.** "This torches more calories and adds new challenge to the muscles of the lower body," says Matthews. (You'll feel it more in your glutes, a.k.a. your rear!)
- **Pedal backwards.** Going forward will tone your hamstrings (the backs of your thighs), but reversing the direction that you pedal will target your quads (the fronts of your thighs). Switch off with each set of three intervals—one forward, one backward, one forward, and so on.
- **Use your arms.** If your machine has the moveable arms, alternate between pushing and pulling motions to increase your calorie burn and work *all* of your upper body muscles.

Fitness Fix:
Find Your Fit Goal

If you're frustrated by continued weight gain or a few pesky pounds you can't seem to shed, your first instinct may be to walk longer or harder, or to up your time on the elliptical machine. What many women don't realize, however, is that strength training is just as crucial as cardio for

When Is the Best Time to Exercise?

"I really boils down to what works for you, regularly *and* consistently," says Matthews. That said, it can pay off to be strategic. Here, the best time to...

- **Form a habit.** Morning! According to one study, 75 percent of morning exercisers stuck with their routines, as compared to only 25 percent of evening exercisers. Plus, "you start your day off with a high burn, and get your energy up and metabolism running," says Jenn Burke, fitness manager for Crunch Gyms in Los Angeles.

- **Boost your brain.** Midday! If you hit a mental roadblock at work, walk away from it—literally. Not only will breaking for a brisk 5-to-10 minute walk relieve stress and boost your mood, but "research shows that midday exercise results in improved mental sharpness, better time management and increased productivity," says Matthews.

- **Try a challenging new workout.** Late afternoon! The next time you're considering trying a new workout (say, a boot camp DVD), do it at 4 P.M or 5 P.M., says Matthews. Your body temperature is at its highest, which studies show will boost your workout. Your muscles are more flexible, your strength is at its peak, and your perceived exertion is low (so exercise feels easier).

losing weight and staying slim. "The more muscle you have, the more metabolically active your body will be—so you'll naturally burn calories at a higher rate," says Cindy Whitmarsh, personal trainer and creator of the UFIT series of fitness DVDs. These mini-workouts are designed so you can strategically strength train in quick spurts, depending on your fitness goals. Try to squeeze in two mini-makeovers that target different muscle groups (for example, one upper body and one lower body) on three non-consecutive days each week, while also working on flexibility and balance (this is key to preventing injuries) twice a week.

MINI-MAKEOVER #6
Tighten Your Arms

Bingo wings, underarm waddle—whatever you call the flab on the back side of your biceps, you want it gone. Luckily, toning this trouble spot is as easy as giving those triceps just a little bit of attention, since they're largely underused in everyday life. A tricep dip is your best start, as it will allow you to build strength quickly.

DO IT: Start with 2 to 3 sets of the Floor Dip; as you get stronger, sub in two to three sets of the Tricep Dips with Leg Lift to continue seeing results.

1. **Floor Dip, p. 255**
2. **Triceps Dip with Leg Lift, p. 256**

MINI-MAKEOVER #7
Flatten Your Stomach

If you want to blast belly fat, this quick mini-workout is designed to strengthen your core and tone your abs long-term. It'll also help you beat bloat, since the Seated Twist increases blood flow to your tummy and stimulates digestion.

DO IT: Repeat this sequence of moves 2 to 3 times.

3. **Toe Taps, p. 256**
4. **Standing Crunch, p. 257**
5. **Seated Twist, p. 257**

MINI-MAKEOVER #8
Firm Your Backside

As you get older, your tissue tends to go a little soft. But because the glutes are your biggest muscle group, that loss of tone can be much more noticeable in your rear. Strengthening the butt muscles and hamstrings, though, can restore some shape to your backside.

DO IT: Start with 10 reps of each move. Eventually, work up to 15, then 20.

6. **Floor Kick, p. 258**
7. **Lying Leg Curl, p. 258**

MINI-MAKEOVER #9
Lose Love Handles

To target that pesky flab that bulges out at your sides, you need moves that hit your abdominal muscles, obliques (the muscles on the side of your stomach) and hips. These exercises do it all.

DO IT: Complete 30 seconds of Crossovers, then do 2 to 3 sets each of the

Side Lift and Twisting Crunch.

8. **Crossovers, p. 259**
9. **Side Lift, p. 259**
10. **Twisting Crunch, p. 260**

MINI-MAKEOVER #10
Strengthen Your Back

"Most things we do in life are forward moving, so we can't forget to strengthen our back to fight gravity," says Whitmarsh. These exercises will also prevent your shoulders from rounding, so you stand tall and strong.

DO IT: Complete 1 set of each move.

11. **Pointers, p. 260**
12. **Scapula Squeeze, p. 261**

MINI-MAKEOVER #11
Shape your legs

Exercising your legs—which are one of your largest muscle groups—is one of the easiest ways to build that lean muscle mass and increase your metabolism. What's more: Strong legs are also a key component of better balance, says Whitmarsh.

DO IT: Complete 2 to 3 sets of each move

13. **Split Squat, p. 261**
14. **Single-Leg Glute Bridge, p. 262**

MINI-MAKEOVER #12
Tone All Over

If you want to get stronger and firmer from head to toe, this one-move makeover is perfect. The exercise, a push-up to a standing jump, works arms, shoulders, chest, back, core and lower body. Bonus: It gets your heart rate up with a short burst of cardio, giving you an anti-aging afterglow.

DO IT: Start with 2 to 3 sets of 5 reps. Progress to 2 to 3 sets of 10 reps.

15. **Beginner's Burpee, p. 262**

MINI-MAKEOVER #13
Improve Your Posture

Slumping adds the appearance of years *and* pounds. So try these three moves for a flat tummy and strong back. Not only will getting stronger help you to stand up straighter (no hunchback down the line!), but you'll also become more aware of your posture—for an instantly anti-aging, slimming effect.

DO IT: Do 2 to 3 sets each of Wall Push-Ups and Scapula Squeeze. Repeat the Modified Plank Hold twice.

16. **Wall Push-Ups, p. 263**

12. **Scapula Squeeze, p. 261**

17. **Modified Plank, p. 263**

MINI-MAKEOVER #14
Improve Your Flexibility

Performing some simple stretches or yoga poses several times a week will prevent the type of stiffness that takes the spring out of your step. You'll also elongate your spine and muscles, for a slimmer, stronger appearance.

DO IT: Go through this sequence of stretches 2 to 4 times.

18. **Forward Bend, p. 264**

19. **Downward Dog, p. 264**

20. **Figure 4, p. 264**

MINI-MAKEOVER #15
Boost Your Balance

You might not think balance is a big deal—yet. But as you get older, your center of gravity shifts, and the number of nerve endings in your feet diminishes. Both of these changes contribute to a little more wobble in your walk, which can lead to clumsiness or falls. Luckily, you can improve your equilibrium with just a few minutes of exercise per week.

DO IT: Repeat each exercise 2 to 4 times, as described.

21. **Warrior 3, p. 265**
22. **Flamingo, p. 266**

SAVINGS TIP!

Four Ways to Slash Fitness Costs

Walking is free, but deals and freebies can help you try new workouts or get gear that makes it easier to work out.

1. Find a free class. Many Pilates or yoga studios offer an introductory class at no charge. You can also ask a friend to bring you along to a group fitness class at her gym—most offer "guest passes" for the same reason.

2. Buy used machines. If you like the elliptical or exercise bike and prefer to work out at home, search Craigslist for secondhand deals—you could save hundreds of dollars. (Just wear comfy clothing so you can test the equipment before you buy.)

3. Score a gym discount. Some clubs tailor a membership if you only use certain facilities, says Meredith Poppler, spokesperson for the International Health, Racquet and Sportsclub Association. Also ask about off-peak discounts. "If the gym is empty between 10 A.M. and 2 P.M., the manager might give special rates for only going then," Poppler says.

4. Go online. YouTube's BeFIT channel (*youtube.com/befit*) offers free videos from fitness experts like Jillian Michaels and Jane Fonda. Most of the routines are 15 minutes or less.

QUICK TIP

Ditch the distraction.
Do you flip through a magazine or watch the news while on a machine at the gym?

"If you want to cut your workout time in half and slim down faster, focus on your body, not the tube," says celebrity trainer Ramona Braganza. "One study found that thinking about the muscles you're using as you work them allows you to use more muscle fibers and build more strength."

Fitness Fix: Make Over Your Day

Between family duties and other responsibilities, there will undoubtedly be days when a workout is not in the cards. That doesn't mean exercise can't happen, though. Even when your schedule is jam-packed, there are tactics to tone up and get your blood pumping. "The research suggests that the activities of daily living, when done with enough intensity, count," says Michael Mantell, a senior consultant in behavioral psychology for the American Council on Exercise. These mini-makeovers will change the way you look at your time—so that every minute is a chance to get fit and feel great.

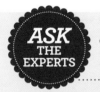

ASK THE EXPERTS
Should I Exercise When I'm Sick?

Do the neck check: If your symptoms are above your neck—you have a stuffy runny nose or a sore throat—moderate exercise like brisk walking is fine, says David Nieman, DrPH, spokesperson for the American College of Sports Medicine. But if you have a fever, deep chest cough or nausea, those below-the-neck signs indicate that what you have is more severe and your body needs more resources to fight it. "Exerting yourself can suppress your immune system, and research shows that exercising heavily with these symptoms can worsen your illness and make it linger longer," says Dr. Nieman.

MINI-MAKEOVER #16
Fine Tune Your Morning

Not sure you'll have time to exercise today? You'll hardly notice these **6 minutes** of strategic activity, which will put you on track for a healthy day.

1 When you wake up... If you shower in the morning, drink some water, then take 3 minutes to cram in a mini-workout that will start your day right:

- 2 min: Do a short burst of cardio, like Beginner's Burpees (See: Exercise #15, p. 262). This gets your blood pumping and metabolism going.
- 15 sec: Rest.
- 45 sec: Cool down and gently stretch your muscles with a relaxing yoga pose. Choose an inversion, like the Forward Bend (See: Exercise #18, p. 264) or Downward Dog (See: Exercise #19, p. 264), to send blood circulating to your face. This can help to give you a glow all day long.

2 As you brush your teeth... You should be brushing for 2 minutes for maximum benefits, so use that time to tone your calves: Press up onto the balls of your feet, using your free hand to hold on to the sink or counter for balance. Stay there for a few seconds, tightening your glutes and abs, then lower down and repeat.

3 While your coffee brews or oatmeal cooks... Grab two soup cans from the cupboard and use them to do simple bicep curls, which will tone your upper arms:

- Start by standing with feet should-width apart and arms at sides, holding one soup can in each hand with palms facing forward.

- Bend your arms at the elbow, curling the cans up to your chest.
- Slowly return to start. Do 10 to 12 reps.

MINI-MAKEOVER #17
Revamp Your Day

Incorporating a little more movement into your workday (especially if you have a desk job) can be life-changing. Not only will sitting less during the day add years to your life, but breaking for a quick stretch or pounding out a 10-minute walk on your lunch break can relieve stress and energize your afternoon.

1 **While you wait in line for coffee...** Pick your left leg up behind you, so that your left toe just barely grazes the ground. Sneakily steady your weight on your right leg. Push your hips back (you'll feel your leg straighten), brace your abdominals (like someone's tightening a belt around your waist) and hold. This improves your balance, posture *and* core muscles. Use it when you're in line for lunch or at the grocery store too.

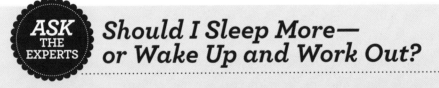

ASK THE EXPERTS *Should I Sleep More— or Wake Up and Work Out?*

As long as you're sleeping for at least 7 hours, it's best to get up and work out, says Robert Oexman, DC, director of the Sleep to Live Institute in Joplin, Maryland. The benefits of exercise outweigh more slumber at this point. But if you were up late and slept less than 7 hours (especially if your total zzz's were under 6 hours), stay in bed. Here's why: Lack of enough quality sleep has been shown to cause shifts in blood glucose levels that increase your appetite and lead to weight gain.

2 On your lunch break... You may go for a walk and reward yourself with lunch afterward, but try flipping your routine. Eat something healthy that you pack from home, then go outside and walk
for 10 to 15 minutes—or climb up and down your building's stairs.
"Studies show that walking right after a meal may help you burn
more fat," says Smith.

3 During your mid-afternoon slump... Stave off the energy dip
that typically happens around 3 P.M. (it affects your muscles, too!)
by practicing good posture while *also* toning your tummy. Wherever you are, sit or stand tall and tighten your stomach by pulling
your belly button in toward your spine and holding for a slow count
to 10. Keep your shoulders back and pelvis relaxed.

MINI-MAKEOVER #18
Refresh Your Evening

You know those days where you feel like all attempts at being healthy
have gone haywire? Use these tactical toning moves to squeeze in some
last-ditch exercise and reset your brain and body. Bonus: By doing even a
little something that's good for your health, you'll feel more accomplished
and at peace when it's time to wind down and go to bed.

1 As you're cooking dinner... Do 10 to 15 "counter push-ups." Stand
about an arm's length away from the counter, place your hands on
the edge and then take a few steps back. Tighten your stomach with
spine straight and bend your elbows as you bring your chest toward
the counter, then push back up. Tip: Don't rush. Take it slowly to
build more muscle.

2 As you talk to a friend on the phone... Multitask with squats (a great toner for your butt, thighs and hips) while you chat. Just lower your body as if you were about to sit down in a chair. Work up to 3 sets of 25 reps per conversation.

3 During your favorite TV show... Use the commercial breaks to strengthen your abs and back. As soon as one starts, get into a Modified Plank (See: p. 263). Try to hold the position through at least two advertisements before getting up.

TRY: Three More Cardio Workouts

Are you on the hunt for a new fitness DVD or dying to try another class at your gym? These workout wonders will give you your most bang for your buck.

1. Kettlebell Training. Some cardio workouts incorporating kettlebells (they're round weights with handles) burn up to 20 calories per minute—that's equivalent to running at a 6-minute-mile pace, says Matthews.

2. Boot Camps. These classes or DVDs pack in high-intensity cardio intervals and strength-training moves that will help you burn fat faster, while also giving you muscle-building benefits you wouldn't get from walking or riding a bike.

3. Zumba. In terms of calorie burn, this fun form of dance tops all of the other popular group fitness classes, according to ACE research. Bonus: Learning choreography and coordinating your brain with your body helps keep your mind sharp!

Exercise Library

1. FLOOR DIP

Tones triceps

A. Sit on the floor with your knees bent and feet flat on the ground. Move your arms behind you about 6 inches and place palms flat on the ground, pointing forward.

B. Bend your elbows as you lean back a few inches. Hold for 2 seconds, then push back up to starting position. Repeat 12 times.

 For added tummy toning, lift your bottom, squeeze your abs and hold for 5 seconds—either before or after the dip.

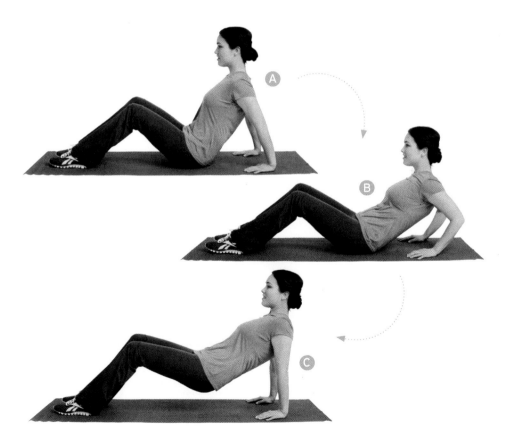

Exercise Library

2. TRICEPS DIP WITH LEG LIFT

A. Sit at edge of a bench (or sturdy chair) with thighs parallel to floor. Lift yourself off bench so you're supported by hands and feet, then raise right leg.
B. Lower body, bending elbows and extending right leg 6 inches to side. Push body back up; bring leg back to center. Do one set of 10 to 20 reps, then repeat with left leg.

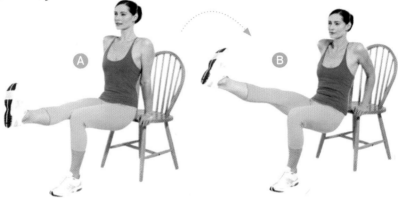

3. TOE TAPS

Relieves shoulder/back tension and tones your tummy

HOW TO: Lie faceup on the foam roller. Bend your legs and lift them toward your chest. Slowly touch your right foot to the ground, then alternate with your left. Do 10 to 20 reps.

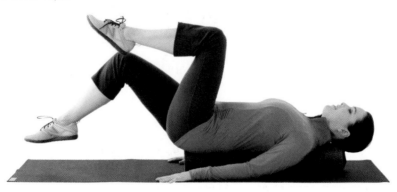

4. STANDING CRUNCH

Tones your abs

A. Stand with feet shoulder-width apart, elbows bent and hands behind head.

B. Bend your left leg and lift your knee across your body as you twist your torso and lower your right elbow toward that knee. Continue alternating sides in a marching motion for 60 seconds.

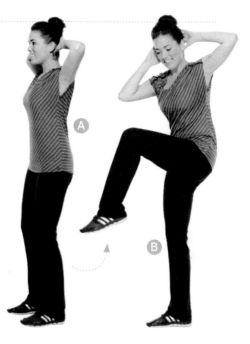

5. SEATED TWIST

Elongates spine and strengthens and stretches core muscles

HOW TO: Sit with legs in front of you. Extend the right leg straight out, flexing the foot. Cross the left foot over the right knee. Lift right arm straight up, then turn torso to the left and place right forearm around left knee. Using your abs and your right arm as leverage, twist torso gently to the left, keeping tailbone on the ground. Inhale and lift spine, exhale and then twist a bit more. Hold for 1 minute, breathing deeply. Release and repeat on the other side.

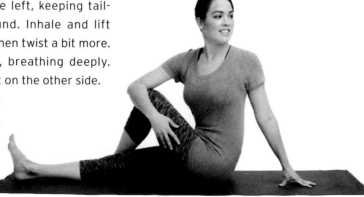

6. FLOOR KICK

Tones rear and legs

A. Start on all fours with your hands and knees on the ground. Lift your leg a few inches off the floor, keeping your knee bent.

B. With the sole of your foot parallel to the ceiling, raise your leg as high as you can. Squeeze your glutes, then return to start. Repeat 10 times, then switch legs.

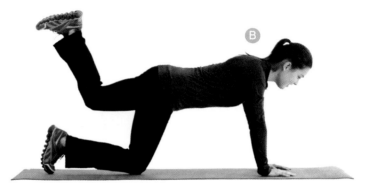

7. LYING LEG CURL

Tones rear and legs

A. Lie facedown with arms at your sides, palms on the floor and legs extended behind you.

B. Keeping your thighs on the ground and arms at your sides, slowly curl your lower legs up toward your bottom, then lower back down. Do 10 reps.

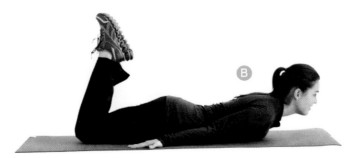

8. CROSSOVERS

Tones tummy and hips

A. Lie on your back with your arms perpendicular to your body. Bend your knees and place your feet flat on the ground.

B. Lower your legs to the left, with upper back on the ground. Return to position A, then repeat to the right. Continue this side-to-side motion for 30 seconds.

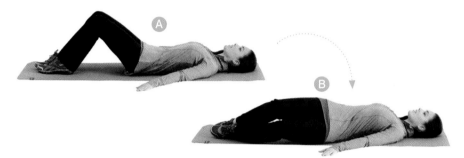

9. SIDE LIFT

A. Lie on mat on your left side, lining up shoulders, hips and knees. Prop head on left hand, with elbow on mat. Place your right hand in front of you to keep you from rolling over. Contract abs.

B. Starting with feet together, lift right leg 6 inches, then lower. (For a challenge, lift both legs off mat about 4 inches, then raise top leg.) Do 10 to 20 reps. Switch sides and repeat.

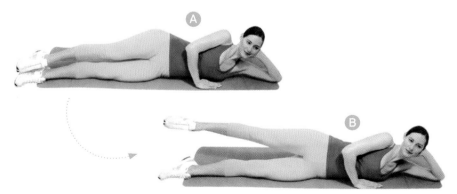

10. TWISTING CRUNCH

A. Lie on your back on mat, feet in air with knees bent at a 90-degree angle. Place hands behind head, keeping elbows wide.

B. Lift shoulders off mat; rotating right shoulder toward outside of left knee as you lower knees slightly to the left. Return to center, and repeat on opposite side. Do 10 to 20 reps.

TIP: If your back arches off the mat, simply place your feet flat on the mat, keeping knees bent, and lower as directed from this position.

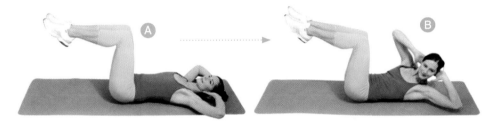

11. POINTERS

Tones arms, back and legs

A. Start on your hands and knees.

B. Extend your left arm and right leg until they are straight and parallel to the ground. Return to the starting position and repeat with opposite limbs. Continue alternating sides for 30 seconds.

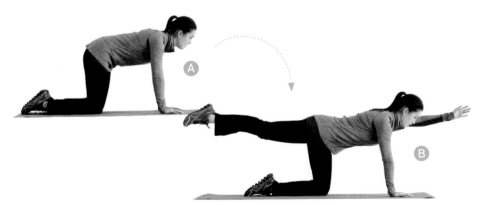

12. SCAPULA SQUEEZE

Tones upper-back muscles and prevents slouching

Stand with feet shoulder-width apart. Bend your elbows and keep arms up, with palms facing out (to form a W with your upper body). Then pull your shoulders back and squeeze your shoulder blades together. Hold for 3 seconds and release. Repeat 10 to 20 times.

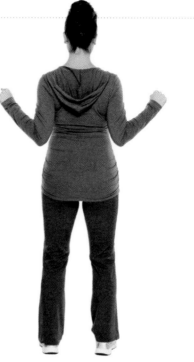

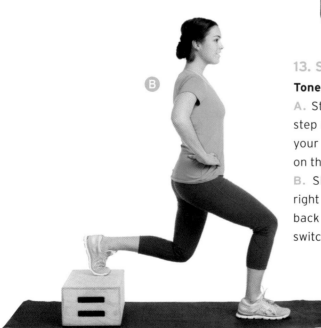

13. SPLIT SQUAT

Tones all lower body muscles

A. Stand about 2 feet away from a step or box, hands on your hips. Lift your left leg back so that your foot is on the step.

B. Slowly bend both knees. Keep right shin straight up and down. Push back to start; repeat 15 times, then switch legs.

14. SINGLE-LEG GLUTE BRIDGE

Tones hamstrings

A. Lie on your back with your arms at your sides. Bend your left knee to 90 degrees, with left foot flat on the floor.

B. Keeping your right leg straight, raise your hips so you create a line from your knee to your shoulder. Hold for 10 seconds. Repeat on other side.

15. BEGINNER'S BURPEE

Works your whole body (arms, shoulders, chest, back, core, lower body, cardio)

A. Stand in front of a table or counter up to 3 feet high. Bend over and place your hands on the top of the ledge, then step your feet back one at a time so your torso forms a straight line. Do a push-up.

B. Walk your feet back in, stand up and raise your arms over your head. Do 5 to 10 reps.

BOOST THE BURN Add a jump when you return to standing, or use a lower surface—like a bench—for your push-up.

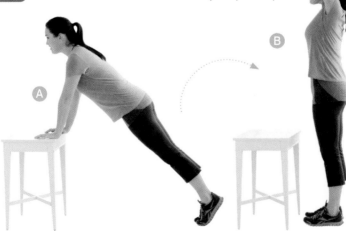

16. WALL PUSH-UPS
Tones chest muscles and keeps your upper body lifted

HOW TO: Stand about 3 feet away from a wall and lean forward, placing your hands shoulder-width apart against the wall. Bend your elbows and bring your chest toward the wall (your heels may come off the floor), then push away until your arms are straight. Repeat 10 to 20 times.

17. MODIFIED PLANK
Tones abdominal and spinal muscles (for a strong torso)

HOW TO: Start on your hands and knees. Place your forearms on the ground with your shoulders over your elbows, and extend your legs. Lower your knees to the ground. Hold for 10 to 30 seconds (or as long as you can without losing form).

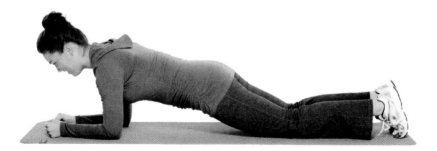

18. FORWARD BEND

Stretches hamstring muscles and lengthens spine

HOW TO: Stand with feet hip-width apart, knees slightly bent and hands on hips. Keep hips directly over knees as you hinge forward at the waist until you're at a 90-degree angle, back flat. Hold there for one slow inhale and exhale, making each breath 5 to 8 seconds, then lower all the way down, allowing gravity to lengthen your back. Touch the ground with your hands, bending knees as much as you need to. Hold for 1 minute total.

FOR A DEEPER STRETCH: Grab your elbows and hang, letting head and neck relax. Hold for 1 minute, breathing in deeply and exhaling slowly. To come up, place hands on hips and stand up.

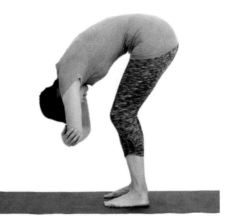

19. DOWNWARD DOG

Stretches and strengthens almost everything, including legs, shoulders, back, arms

HOW TO: Start standing up and fold forward, knees bent. Place hands on the ground with palms flat and fingers forward. Walk feet back 3 to 4 feet until legs are straight (or almost straight), back flat, bottom toward ceiling. Keep your gaze between ankles to relax your neck, and press heels toward the mat to stretch the back of legs. Hold the position for 5 to 10 deep inhales and exhales.

20. FIGURE 4

Loosens up tight hip muscles (a cause of back pain)

HOW TO: Lie with back flat on the ground, legs extended. Draw your left knee to your chest and hold it there for a breath or two. Bend your right leg so the knee is

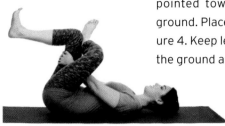

pointed toward ceiling and right foot is on the ground. Place left ankle on right knee to create a figure 4. Keep left foot flexed and push tailbone toward the ground as you gently pull your right knee toward your chest with your hands. Hold for 1 minute as you inhale and exhale. Repeat on the other side.

21. WARRIOR 3

Works your core and improves balance

HOW TO: Stand a few feet away from a wall, place your hands flat against it and lean into the wall slightly. Lift your left leg a few feet off the ground behind you. Contract your stomach muscles and hold this position for 30 seconds. Switch legs and hold for another 30 seconds.

 TO BOOST THE BURN Lower your arms on the wall and lift your leg higher. Your body should make a T shape.

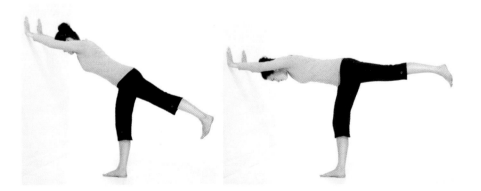

Exercise Library

22. FLAMINGO

Stretches and strengthens leg/core muscles and improves balance

A. Stand with your feet shoulder-width apart. Lift your right leg behind you, knee bent, balancing on your left leg. Extend your left arm up by your head and grasp right foot with right hand.

B. Gently pull up on your right leg and hinge forward. Go as far as you can while staying balanced, then straighten back up. Lower your foot; repeat with your left leg.

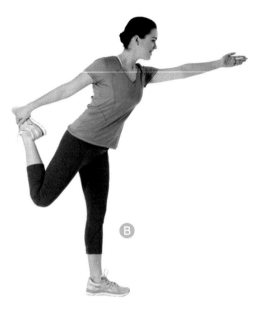

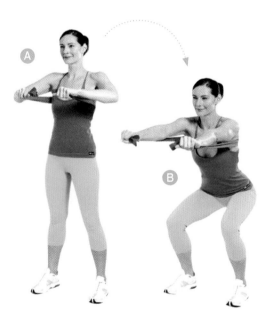

23. SQUAT WITH CHEST PRESS

A. Stand with feet shoulder-width apart. Wrap band around shoulder blades and hold an end in each hand, arms at chest level, elbows out.

B. Lower body into a squat, sitting back into heels with knees over ankles, until thighs are nearly parallel to ground. At the same time, press arms straight out in front of you at chest height. Do 8 to 10 reps.

The Quickie Guide
to Fitness

If you do nothing else, try one or all of these tips for better fitness.

1. Move Every Day Your metabolism is slowing, so you need to clock at least 30 minutes of physical activity daily. (Walking counts!) Bonus: It'll do wonders for your mood too.

2. Reboot Your Cardio Three times a week, make sure you up the intensity with a 20-minute workout that incorporates intervals (switching up speeds) and climbs (using hills, steps or inclines). These factors help you pack in more of a burn.

3. Get Strong It's not just about toning up: When you build lean muscle mass, you boost your metabolism, improve your posture (an instant anti-ager!) and blast fat faster. That's why strength training three times a week is a must.

4. Tuck Your Tummy A simple rule: If you always remember to keep your abs tight, you can turn any type of exercise—from walking to mopping floors—into a core-firming multitasker.

5. Engage Your Brain Exercise will keep your mind sharp. So make it a point to include activities that challenge you to react (like tennis), learn complex movements (like Zumba) or change directions (like a walking workout with side-stepping).

6. Find Balance Doing a little bit of balance training now (just standing on one leg counts!) will pay you back later, when your center of gravity shifts. Plus it makes you feel steadier and more confident when you try different workouts, like dance.

7. Stretch it Out Working on your flexibility a few times a week is like a youth elixir. You nix stiffness and increase your energy, plus your posture improves.

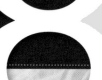

Sleep Better Tonight

8

Easy tweaks to help you get the rest you need to look and feel amazing

Set Yourself Up to Snooze
Get your body, brain and bedroom ready for deep, restorative sleep

Target Your Sleep Issue
What's keeping you up—and how to fix it

66 When I'm tired, I rest. I say, 'I can't be superwoman today.'" —*Jada Pinkett Smith*

Y ou used to fall asleep as soon as your head hit the pillow. Now your brain races and your body can't seem to get comfortable. "We spend so much time raising children, having careers and taking care of the different generations in our families," says Susie Esther, MD, a Charlotte-based sleep specialist and spokesperson for the American Academy of Sleep Medicine. "Sleep is not a priority."

But it pays to make it one. Research has linked sleep deprivation to everything from diabetes to heart disease to cancer, and doctors believe that robbing your body of shut-eye knocks your hormones—ones that control everything from weight to mood to metabolism—out of whack. Give yourself enough zzz's, though, and the consequences can be equally life-changing—in a more positive direction.

- **Sleep can slim you.** Studies show that people who sleep more weigh less, probably because you have more energy to exercise and you're less likely to crave foods high in fat and sugar.

- **Sleep may save your skin.** "When you sleep, there's a boost of blood flow to skin, which prompts cells to turn over eight times faster than during the day," says David E. Bank, MD, a dermatologist in Mount Kisco, New York. Getting fewer than 6 hours increases the stress hormone cortisol, which slows collagen.

- **Sleep can make you happier.** One night of lousy sleep makes you grouchy, but there's also a huge overlap between consistently poor sleep and mood disorders. Research suggests that insomniacs may be up to 10 times more likely to experience depression, and 17 times more likely to suffer from anxiety.

There are a number of factors that could be keeping you from getting the deep, restorative sleep you need. Some are easily fixable (like your pre-bed routine or caffeine habit), while others are a result of the inevitable hormonal changes that happen as you move toward menopause. "As we get older, we don't sleep as efficiently," says Dr. Esther. "So we need to put extra effort into working on the habits that will help."

How to use this chapter

For women, sleep issues come in many forms—from having trouble falling asleep, to rousing with hot flashes, to thinking you slept OK but not waking up refreshed. The advice in this chapter is divided into two parts:

- **Set Yourself Up to Snooze** Is your bedtime too early? Could the temperature of your room be waking you up at night? Here you'll find mistakes you may be making, and the lifestyle changes that will put you on track for better sleep every night.

- **Target Your Sleep Issue** Whether you lie in bed worrying every night or wake up exhausted, these mini-makeovers will help you cope in the moment—and find the root cause of your most frustrating issue.

How Sleep Works

Knowing what happens when you sleep will help you understand why quantity (total time) and quality (how well you sleep through the night) count. Sleep consists of two different states, forming a roughly 90-minute cycle that repeats, on average, five times over the course of the night. Fun fact: Most people awaken for about 20 to 30 seconds at the end of each cycle, then fall back to sleep. (This is normal! And about 90 percent of people never even remember it, says Michael Breus, PhD, author of *The Sleep Doctor's Diet Plan*.)

1 **NREM (non-rapid eye movement) Sleep:**
- Stage 1: Very light sleep—you're somewhere between being asleep and awake. (Waking from this stage can make you feel like you haven't slept.)
- Stage 2: Sleep starts—your body temperature drops, and breathing and heart rate become regular.
- Stages 3 to 4: Deep, restorative sleep—your muscles relax even more, your breathing becomes slow and rhythmic, and your body tissues repair themselves. Energy is restored, and hormones that regulate growth and appetite are released. (If roused, you may feel disoriented.)

2 **REM (rapid eye movement) Sleep:** Your muscles relax and become immobile, while your heart rate speeds up and breathing becomes rapid and shallow. This is the period of heightened brain activity—when dreaming occurs and memories are processed. (If you remember your dreams, you're likely waking up during this state.)

The Bottom Line: When you wake up in the middle of the night, you restart the sleep cycle all over again. If sleep is cut short, you miss cycles all together. Either way, you're robbing yourself of completing all the phases needed to repair muscles and skin, solidify memories and release hormones that help control hunger.

Set Yourself Up to Snooze

Good sleep starts with good habits, and here's why: Even if you're prone to some very specific sleep-killers—like before-bed worry or nighttime heartburn—changing what you do during the day and where you sleep at night will help you keep the consistent schedule that calms your mind and drives your body to sleep through disruptions. So consider these first three mini-makeovers your starting point: Together, they'll correct the mistakes you don't even know you're making.

MINI-MAKEOVER #1
Reset Your Sleep Schedule

The first question on your mind is surely this one: How much sleep do I really need? While doctors say that most women typically require between 7 to 8 hours, not everyone will fall in that range—and it pays to figure out what works best for you. "There is such a thing as too much sleep, and there is such a thing as too little sleep," says Dr. Breus, who adds that excessive sleep can make you feel sluggish and foggy, just like sleep deprivation. "What you're looking for is a balance."

So ask yourself: What's your morning usually like—do you typically hop out of bed, or is rousing yourself a daily struggle? "If you feel refreshed and ready to meet the day within a minute or two of waking up, then that's how much sleep you need," says Dr. Breus. Otherwise, you might want to consider shifting your sleep schedule. Once you find your sweet spot and stick to it, you'll sleep more soundly and feel more refreshed. Here's how to do it:

1 **Start with your wakeup time.** This is almost always predetermined by your life demands, so choose a reasonable time that you feel confident you can stick to seven days a week.

2 **Calculate your bedtime.** To start, count back seven-and-a-half hours. For example, if your wake time is 6:30 A.M., you should aim to go to sleep at 11 P.M.

3 **Try it out for five days.** Set yourself up for the best sleep possible (See: Tweak Your Daily Routine, p. 275), then see what your mornings feel like:

- Are you waking up ahead of your alarm? The next night, try pushing your bedtime a half hour later, to 11:30 P.M.
- Do you hit the snooze button? Shift that bedtime up a half hour, to 10:30 P.M., and see how that feels.

Experiment until you start waking up refreshed at your desired time.

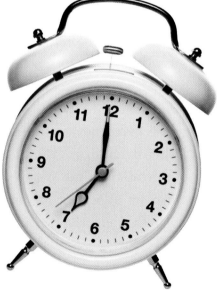

MINI-MAKEOVER #2
Tweak Your Daily Routine

Getting a good night's sleep is about more than hitting your target bedtime. It starts as soon as you wake up that morning, because every little habit—from what you eat and drink to when you exercise and watch TV—can impact your sleep. Here's a sample day that shows what you can do to get the best sleep possible. Adjust it for your own personal wakeup and sleep times.

6:30 A.M. Skip the snooze button

It's tempting to turn over and squeeze in an extra 10 to 15 minutes of shut-eye when your alarm goes off, but doing so can actually make you *more* tired. "You spend so much energy going back to sleep and waking up again that you don't get any additional deep sleep," says Kathryn Lee, RN, PhD, professor and associate dean for research at the University of California San Francisco School of Nursing. Instead, throw open the shades or turn on the lights. Darkness prompts your body to produce more melatonin, a hormone that helps you feel sleepy, but brightness will give you an instant lift. And if you do it every morning, you can train your body to produce less melatonin overall.

7 A.M. Exercise

Physical activity in the morning may decrease levels of stress hormones, making it easier for your body to wind down later, says Scott Collier, PhD, director of the Vascular Biology and Autonomic Studies Laboratory at Appalachian State University. In one study, people who did 30 minutes of moderate exercise at 7 A.M. (compared with 1 P.M. and 7 P.M.) significantly improved their sleep quality that night, spending 75 percent more time in deep sleep.

SLEEP BETTER

11 A.M. Take a breathing break

If you don't take time to stop during the day, falling asleep is harder. Why? "When you finally try, you lie awake thinking about all of the things you haven't had a moment to ponder," says Diane Renz, LPC, a psychotherapist in Boulder, Colorado. It's kind of like slamming on the brakes of a fast-moving car and all of the junk in the back flying forward. At least twice a day, close your eyes and take three slow, deep breaths.

1 P.M. to 2 P.M. Reduce caffeine intake

"Caffeine is a stimulant that lasts in your system for 4 to 7 hours," says Lawrence Epstein, MD, an instructor at Harvard Medical School. Cutting caffeine out in the afternoon won't just let the stimulating effects

ASK THE EXPERTS *What If I'm a Night Owl?*

Do you feel most alert and productive in the evening—then you can't seem to wind down until well after your ideal bedtime? Sleep is regulated by our internal body clock, or "circadian rhythm." If you want to go to bed earlier but your body won't cooperate, you may need to reset your inner clock. The easiest way to do it: Set your alarm for the desired time and put it across the room, and when you wake up, open the blinds immediately. Exposure to daylight shifts your brain into daytime mode, which will ultimately help with that sleep/wake balance once it's time to go to bed. (Is it still dark out? Invest in a light box or dawn stimulator, which mimics outdoor light—about $60 and up at *amazon.com*.) If that still doesn't help—and you've tried the tips in Mini-Makeovers 2 and 3—talk to your doctor about a melatonin supplement. It's the hormone that brings on sleepiness, and a low dose (no more than 1.5 milligrams) taken 5 to 6 hours before your desired bedtime could help you get back on track, says Lisa Shives, MD, a Chicago-based sleep specialist and medical expert for *SleepBetter.org*.

wear off before your bedtime, but it will also help you keep your caffeine intake under 250 milligrams a day, which is the amount experts say most women can handle without sleep-wrecking effects. Remember, coffee (95 milligrams per cup) isn't the only culprit: Tea (40 milligrams per cup), chocolate (25 milligrams per 1.45 ounce) and diet cola (47 milligrams per can) also contain levels that can affect your sleep.

3 P.M. Go outside

Getting out in natural afternoon light (30 minutes is ideal—even if it's cloudy) not only energizes you, but it also helps reset your circadian rhythm so you'll wind down easier when bedtime rolls around, says Donna Arand, PhD, clinical director of the Kettering Sleep Disorders Center in Dayton, Ohio. If you can't exercise in the A.M., use this time to squeeze in a brisk walk.

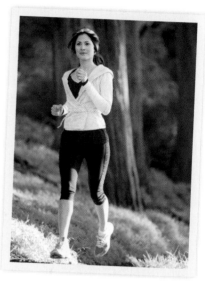

7 P.M. Eat dinner earlier

Your body needs at least 2 hours (3 for a heavy meal) to fully digest food. Also consider what you're eating and drinking. Avoid foods that trigger heartburn like chocolate; garlic; onions; fatty, spicy, greasy or fried foods; acidic foods like citrus or tomatoes; and alcohol. "Alcohol makes you sleepy at first, but causes you to wake up as it wears off," says Nancy Collop, MD, director of the Emory Sleep Program.

10 P.M. Have a protein-carb snack

Eating this combo an hour before bedtime helps. Your brain needs the protein to produce melatonin and serotonin, chemicals important for sleep, and the carbs help your body absorb the protein, says Dr. Lee.

A healthy snack option: 1 Tablespoon hummus in a mini whole-wheat pita. (See: Bonus Food Fix, *below.*)

10:15 P.M. Unplug

About 45 minutes to one hour before bed, turn off the TV, power down your computer and put your iPad away too. Surfing the Internet and reading emails stimulates your nervous system, making it harder to unwind, plus the short-wave blue light emitted by all of these devices' screens sends a message to your body that says, *Hey! More daylight! Let's stay up and get stuff done.* If you like to read before bed,

---

BONUS FOOD FIX
Eat and Drink for Better Sleep

These snacks and drinks can make for a more restful slumber.

1. The Doze Bowl The classic sleep prescription of a small bowl of cereal and milk has scientific backing. The combination of protein and carbs triggers your brain to produce serotonin, its sleep-inducing chemical. (Not actually hungry? Try a cup of warm milk, which might help bring on sleepiness too.)

2. Cherry Pick Tart cherry juice is practically a melatonin cocktail. To score the benefits, drink an 8-ounce glass (or 2 Tablespoons of tart cherry juice concentrate in 8 ounces of water) twice a day.

3. Trail-Off Mix Make a trail mix with pumpkin seeds. In addition to the sleep-promoting chemicle tryptophan, they contain zinc, which helps convert tryptophan to slumber-inducing serotonin. For an even bigger boost of these chemicals, mix in carb-rich dried fruit, like apples, apricots or blueberries.

4. Get-Tired Tea Sip a cup of chamomile tea 30 to 45 minutes before bedtime. It has a gentle tranquilizing effect, which can help to calm your mind.

e-readers with "e-ink" displays are better options (they don't give off blue light), but you can also adjust the settings on your tablet to minimize brightness. (In iPad's iBooks app, for example, choose the "Night Theme," which displays white text on a black screen.)

10:30 P.M. Begin your wind-down routine

Thirty minutes before bed is the ideal time to start moving into bedtime-mode. "A lot of sleep disturbance happens because we don't give our bodies a chance to transition from a fast-paced day," says Dr. Renz. This can be as simple as taking off your makeup and washing your face under dim lights, but if you've been having trouble falling asleep, try a hot shower. "Hot water raises your core body temperature, which increases muscle relaxation," says Dr. Breus.

11 P.M. Get into bed, breathe and stretch

Taking a few deep breaths and doing a light 30-second stretch will help you relax once you're under the sheets, says Dr. Collop. Try sitting up and reaching toward your toes or getting into child's pose: Kneel, sit back on your heels, then bend forward, resting your torso on your thighs. Don't stress if it takes a little while to fall asleep— up to 20 minutes is normal.

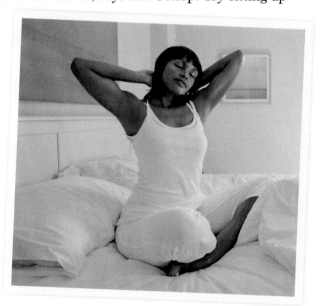

MINI-MAKEOVER #3
Prime Your Bedroom

Sleep doctors have a fancy name for your bedroom—they call it your "sleep environment"—and say that even the tiniest variables can upset your slumber. (You should be like a bear hibernating in a cave, where it's cool, dark and quiet!) So take a look around and check these key factors:

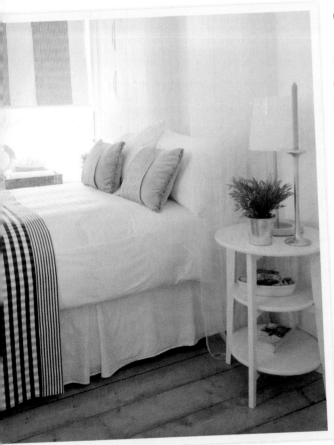

1 THE TEMPERATURE It's more comfortable to sleep in a cool room, especially if you're dealing with hormonal changes and hot flashes. Experts say 67°F to 70°F is ideal, but you don't want it to be too cold. Experiment to find your just-right temperature, and set the thermostat about an hour before bed so your room has time to cool down.

2 THE WINDOWS "Light is probably the biggest factor that will cause problems with sleep," says Dr. Breus. Try blackout shades or curtains. They'll block morning sunshine and help you stick to a consistent snooze schedule year-round, which is key to deeper, more restorative sleep.

3 YOUR PILLOW The wrong pillow can cause neck pain, so try sleeping with a single pillow that comfortably supports your head. Foam pillows offer the most support, and consider how you sleep: A back sleeper needs a thinner pillow, while a side sleeper needs something firmer. A stomach sleeper can choose a thin one or skip it. (Many brands label their pillows by sleep position.)

QUICK TIP
Spritz pillows with jasmine.
This soothing scent can trigger relaxation. To make a DIY linen spray: Add 6 drops jasmine essential oil to 4 ounces water.

4 THE MATTRESS Over time, your body wears down your mattress, making it less supportive (especially if you always sleep in the exact same spot). If you've owned your mattress for more than five years and you're waking up with new aches and pains or noticing it has big indentations, it might be time to go shopping. Otherwise, you can keep your mattress for up to 10 years, and slow down damage by flipping or rotating it every 6 months.

5 YOUR SHEETS Many women wake up drenched in sweat, thanks to the hormonal changes before and during menopause. Linens with a lower thread count (a looser weave allows more heat to escape) or made of moisture-wicking fabric (often labeled "wicking," "performance" or "temperature balance") can help you reduce your body temperature and get sweat-free sleep (bedding starts at $49; *sheex.com*).

6 THE CLUTTER If you're the type of person who gets stressed out by a mess, seeing overflowing piles of clothes or other disarray will make it harder for you to relax and fall asleep. So take 5 minutes to tidy up, and close any open closets or drawers.

SLEEP BETTER

7 YOUR DOG OR CAT A survey by the National Sleep Foundation found that 17 percent of women woke up because of pets moving around or making noise. If you can't bear to banish your furry friend from the bedroom, set up a sleeping area next to the bed.

8 YOUR ALARM CLOCK The light from a digital clock can make the room too bright. The simple fix: Put a towel over the numbers at night. (For more on how alarm clocks affect your sleep, See: Wake Up the Right Way, p. 291.)

9 YOUR CELL PHONE Charge your devices out of reach in the living room or kitchen so you're not tempted to scan social media or browse headlines, which can be stress-inducing. If you must keep your phone bedside, place it facedown (even the smallest amount of light stimulates your nervous system and can disrupt your sleep) and turn off smartphone notifications. For example, iPhones have a "Do Not Disturb" option in settings, which will quiet all alerts.

10 THE NOISE LEVEL Even if you don't think police sirens, car horns or your husband's snores are disrupting your sleep, they might be. Earplugs can help, but you might also want to invest in a white-noise machine, says Dr. Lee. These small, tabletop devices ($20 and up; *amazon.com*) mask distracting sounds in a soothing way, so your brain isn't stimulated as you begin to fall asleep.

11 YOUR LAMP It's important to shift from harsh overhead lighting to a dim glow at least 45 minutes before bed, so put a soft lamp on your bedside table. And if you already have one, check the bulb: You want no more than 45 watts to help you transition into bedtime mode, says Dr. Breus.

Is Your Husband Keeping You Up?

You can't exactly boot him from the bedroom (as you would your smartphone), but there are ways to work out why he's causing you to be awake. Try these tricks.

SLEEP-ZAPPER #1: His Snoring
If you are like 41 percent of women, you are convinced your partner's snoring is what's keeping you from getting a good night's rest.
THE FIX: Attack the issue from both sides. Tell him you'll try earplugs or a white noise machine (See: The Noise Level, p. 282) and stop complaining if *he* agrees to try sleeping on his side and make an appointment with his doctor. (To ease the process, buy him a no-snore pillow, which helps position the head to open up the airways.)

SLEEP-ZAPPER #2: You Hash Out Problems Before Bed
Many couples are so busy all day that they don't have a time to catch up until they climb under the covers. But tackling tough issues right before bed will make your brain hyperalert.
THE FIX: Set a talk time. Tell your husband this bad habit is keeping you up, then make it a point to have a designated time to discuss difficult topics—a pre-dinner conversation or post-dinner walk will still give you time to wind down afterward.

SLEEP-ZAPPER #3: He Gets Up at the Crack of Dawn
Your husband is a lark; you're more of an owl. He flips on a light to find his shoes, and boom—you're wide awake before your body is actually ready.
THE FIX: Plan ahead. Ask him to set out his clothes each night in another room, and keep a small flashlight on his nightstand that will help him see what he needs to see without creating a room-brightening glow. If your sleep still doesn't improve, you can also prep before bed by investing in a sleep mask and earplugs.

What's Keeping You Up— And How to Fix It

Let's say you've been trying to do everything right—you exercise every morning, drink decaf, and turn off your phone at 9 P.M.—but you're still struggling. What can you do? Whether your biggest complaint is lying awake with a head full of worry, or tossing and turning because you just can't seem to get comfortable, there are ways to cope in the moment—and fix your problem for good.

MINI-MAKEOVER #4
Fall Asleep (or Back to Sleep) Faster

For many women in their 30s and beyond, the main sleep issue is this: *No matter how drained I am, I spend half the night staring at the ceiling!* Some experience this sleeplessness as soon as they get into bed; others drift off initially, only to wake up in the middle of the night or early morning. So what can you do? Should you count sheep? Take a sleep aid? It depends on how long you've been struggling. Falling asleep can take up to 20 minutes, says Kathy Gromer, MD, a sleep medicine specialist at the Minnesota Sleep Institute in Minneapolis. So don't expect to drift off the second your head hits the pillow (if you do, it actually means you're sleep-deprived!). Otherwise, follow this advice, which can help you doze off—or fall back to sleep—when your brain feels wide awake.

 Coax Yourself to Sleep

It can be a vicious cycle: Your body and its inner clock are set up for sleep, but you're so fixated on the items you forgot to tick off your to-do list that your brain races you right past that golden opportunity to doze off. Then, once you realize how long you've been lying there, you start to worry about not being able to sleep—and the anxiety escalates. Sound familiar? It's OK. If it's only a once-in-a-while problem, you can distract your brain and lull your body back to sleep mode. Here's your course of action:

- **FIRST: Count backward from 300.** The trick: Do it by multiples of three (300, 297, 294, and so on). "I know it sounds crazy, but, it works really well—I promise," says Dr. Breus. "It's mathematically so complicated that you can't think of anything else, and it's so doggone boring that you're out like a light."

- **IF THAT DOESN'T WORK: Get out of bed.** Most sleep docs say you shouldn't stay in bed for more than 20 minutes, but Dr. Shives has her own rule: "If you're getting annoyed or anxious, don't keep lying there," she says. "Hop out and break the cycle." She advises that you leave the room without flipping on the lights (keep a mini flashlight on your nightstand), then sit quietly in a comfy chair and distract yourself with something soothing, like soft music or an audiobook. And "avoid doing things like paperwork, dishes or folding laundry," adds Dr. Esther. "That rewards you for not sleeping, because work is getting done." Sit there until you finally feel sleepy, then go back to bed.

- **YOUR LAST RESORT: Use a sleep aid.** If drowsiness never sets in, try a sleep aid (don't look at a clock—just use your judgment). Valerian root is a natural supplement that prompts your brain to produce neurotransmitters that make you sleepy, says Dr. Breus. Be careful, though—it makes you *very* tired.

Never take the recommended dose (500 milligrams) less than 4 hours before your alarm goes off. You can also try an over-the-counter sleep aid, like ZzzQuil, or Benadryl (the active ingredient—an antihistamine called Diphenhydramine HCL—is the same, says Dr. Esther, and these bring on sleep without the added pain relievers and cough medicines in other nighttime meds, like Nyquil or Tylenol PM). "Just beware that these OTC meds often cause dry mouth and next-day grogginess—that's why they're a last resort and should only be used occasionally," she adds.

Change Your Nighttime Routine

If your problem continues more than a week, be sure that you're doing all you can to correct bad sleep habits and ensure that your body and brain have a chance to wind down in the evening. (See:

Last Night Was Rough— Should I Take a Nap?

When you aren't getting enough zzz's at night, it's tempting to try to steal a few minutes of shut-eye during the day. And while a short nap (15 to 30 minutes) has restorative benefits, resting for longer can interfere with the quality of your nighttime sleep. "Your body is only programmed to accept about 8 hours of sleep a day, so if you take a two-hour nap, that's automatically going to reduce your nightly sleep to about 6 hours," explains Thomas Roth, PhD, director of the Henry Ford Sleep Disorders and Research Center in Detroit. And the closer to bedtime you nap, the harder it will be to fall asleep at night. To stay on track with your normal sleep schedule (which is more important in the long run), limit your mini snoozes to a late-morning or early-afternoon nap, and try to go to bed no earlier than an hour before your normal bedtime.

Tweak Your Daily Routine, p. 275) And if it's anxiety that's keeping you up? Try adding one of these little mental exercises to your evening ritual:

- **Give yourself "worry time."** This could help to quiet your racing brain come bedtime, says Dr. Esther. Post-dinner is ideal timing, so after you finish putting away the dishes, take out a notebook and answer the question, *What am I anxious about?* Make two columns: One for the concern, and one for what you're going to do about it. Sometimes there's nothing you can do, and that's OK. Simply writing down your worries defines them, which makes you feel like you have some control, while shutting the notebook and putting them aside offers you closure.

- **Rehash your "I did" list.** A little later (like when you're winding down with a warm shower), go over all of the things you did that day in your head, starting with the end and working backward. This will give you peace of mind, plus a relaxing sense of accomplishment.

- **Count your blessings.** Whether you actually write them down in a gratitude journal or simply recite them in your head, taking 2 minutes to focus on the positive aspects of the day—the moment you enjoyed most, or what made you laugh the hardest—can calm your anxiety before bed. Experts say the more descriptive and specific you are about the things that make you thankful, the more happiness and calm you'll gain (think: "a delicious dinner at my favorite restaurant with my best friend," not "food on my plate").

These are simple tactics that you can use on a daily basis to prevent night-time anxiety. However, if your problem lasts two weeks or more, you may need professional help to get you back on track. See your doctor or a sleep specialist to discuss lifestyle changes or prescription medication.

MINI-MAKEOVER #5
Get Comfortable in Bed

You toss, turn, kick your legs around, move your arms—but no matter what you do, it doesn't feel right. Why are some nights (or all nights) so fidgety? There could be several reasons for your restlessness, but some trial and error can help you get to the root cause of your physical discomfort.

FIX IT FAST | **Ease Stiffness and Tweak How You Sleep**

If you can't get comfortable in bed, "your sleep position and pillows could be interfering with your sleep quality, especially if you have back pain during the day, " says Erik St. Louis, MD, an associate professor of neurology at Mayo Clinic College of Medicine. Muscle stiffness or cramps could be another culprit. A few simple tweaks to your pre-bed routine—and how you sleep—can make a big difference. Try this tonight:

1 **BEFORE BED: Relax your muscles.** Take a warm bath, then rub on lotion in circular motions with medium pressure. When you get to a spot that's especially tense, like your neck, press down with your fingertips for 10 seconds. This draws blood flow to the area to promote healing and relaxation.

2 **AT BEDTIME: Find the right position.** Dr. St. Louis suggests these little changes, which could offer big relief:

- **If you're a side sleeper,** try putting a pillow between your knees and thighs to keep your spine straight.

- **If you're a back sleeper,** try placing a flat pillow under your knees or a small, rolled towel under the small of your back.

- **If you're a stomach sleeper,** place a pillow under your pelvis and lower abdomen and use just a thin cushion under the face.

3 IN TENSE MOMENTS: Stretch. "Many people don't realize that stiffness in their joints is causing them to wake up, but you can stretch out while you're lying in your bed," says Dr. Breus. He recommends a figure-4 stretch: Take one leg, cross it over the other bent knee, then bring that knee toward you, so you're making a number *4*. Hold for 10 seconds, then repeat on the other side. "That pulls out your glutes and lower back, which makes sleeping more comfortable," says Dr. Breus.

QUICK TIP

Stop night pain. Don't try to sleep off a headache or cramps. Without treating the pain first, you may wake up throughout the night. Take an over-the-counter painkiller at least 30 minutes before bed (just avoid those containing caffeine so you'll snooze soundly).

Talk to Your Doctor

If you've been plagued by pain, stiffness or restlessness for more than two weeks, discuss the problem with your doctor. Your muscle cramps may be caused by dehydration or an electrolyte imbalance (simply drinking more water can help), or you might need a stronger anti-inflammatory to help ease sore joints. You'll also want to rule out something called Restless Legs Syndrome (RLS), which is a nerve disorder that occurs in about 5 percent of the population. It's characterized by what you might describe as a "creepy crawly" feeling in your legs and—because it's linked to low iron levels—becomes more common as women get older. While massages, relaxation exercises, regular workouts and restoring iron in your diet can help, your doctor may suggest a prescription drug. "It's a sleep doctor's favorite thing to treat, because it's such an easy fix," says Dr. Esther. "The medications are very effective."

SLEEP BETTER

MINI-MAKEOVER #6
Start the Day Refreshed

Do you have difficulty waking up, and—even when you finally do manage to drag your body out of bed—feel like your brain is on a 4-hour delay? Experts call this grogginess and lingering fatigue "sleep inertia," and in one study at the University of Colorado at Boulder, those who awakened with it following 8 hours of sound slumber were more mentally impaired than they would be after 24 hours of sleep deprivation.

Here's why it happens: When you first go to bed, you usually enter light sleep, then deep sleep, then dreaming (REM) sleep. Together, they form a complete cycle that lasts about 90 minutes and repeats four to six times over the course of a night (See: How Sleep Works, p. 272). And in the hour before you're set to wake up, the body prepares itself for the day and sleep gradually becomes lighter. Awaken before you're ready,

---

ASK THE EXPERTS

Can Medications Be Disrupting My Sleep?

Yes, your medicine cabinet may be lined with stimulants. "Several types of prescription drugs, ranging from cardiac drugs that regulate blood pressure to decongestants for the common cold, can aggravate or worsen insomnia," says Dr. St. Louis. Certain asthma medications and antidepressants also fall into the category of meds that inhibit asleep. Of course, this doesn't mean you should ditch your prescription; just be sure to talk to your doctor if sleep issues develop. The solution may be as simple as taking the medications earlier in the day or switching to a different prescription. And if you take a multivitamin, consider downing that in the a.m. hours too. Vitamins like B_6 and B_{12} are involved in nerve and blood cell function as well as energy metabolism, so they can easily disrupt sleep.

though—*especially* during a deep sleep stage—and you'll start your day feeling beat.

 Wake Up the Right Way

Certain A.M. habits can interrupt your natural sleep cycle and zap your energy from the get-go. So to infuse your day with more oomph from the very start, give this expert-approved advice a try:

Consider a Smarter Wake-up Call

As you sleep, your body builds up its supply of a hormone called cortisol, which is released throughout the day to give you energy. But if your alarm blares like a foghorn, you wake up panicked and zap those cortisol stores right away. So switch to an alarm that uses soft sounds or soothing music to coax you (not jerk you) awake, like:

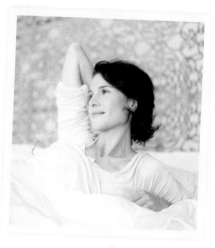

- **The Gentle Alarm app** ($3.99; iTunes). Developed by a neurologist, it slowly brings you out of REM sleep, your final stage.

- **Homedics SoundSpa Autoset Clock Radio** ($29.26; *7yearsyounger.com/shop*) Choose your wakeup call from six nature sounds. As an added value, it's also a white noise machine, which will help you drown out your husband's snores at night.

 Shift Your Sleep Schedule and Check Snoring

If you time your bedtime right, you might not even need an alarm, and you can awake more naturally—or at least from your lightest sleep stage—to avoid extreme fatigue. (For advice on how to find your ideal bedtime and make sure you're getting enough rest, See: Reset Your Sleep Schedule, p. 273.) But you might also want to ask your partner if you've been snoring or run a recorder one night to see for yourself. That's because another common cause of daytime drowsiness is something called obstructive sleep apnea (OSA), a condition that causes your breathing to stop periodically—sometimes for a minute or longer— throughout the night. (You may wake hundreds of times to restart it without ever knowing, which is why next-day sleepiness is often a surprise.) Sleep apnea's major symptom is loud snoring, but you might also notice a dry mouth or sore throat in the morning. If you suspect you're suffering from sleep apnea, here's what you can do about it:

- **Lose weight.** About 65 percent of people who have sleep apnea are overweight or obese. The condition can contribute to—or be a consequence of—extra pounds. Slimming down often improves symptoms and may even cure obstructive breathing.

- **Change your position.** If you're a back sleeper, try sleeping on your side. It can make breathing easier. One way to keep from rolling back again: Place a tennis ball in a sock, then pin the sock to the back of your PJs. It may seem like a weird trick but it works!

- **See your doctor.** Even if your bedmate hasn't said you've been snoring, go in for a checkup. If you have sleep apnea, you may need a continuous positive airway pressure (CPAP) machine. It works by not allowing the soft tissue in your throat to collapse and stop your breathing.

Quickie Guide to Better Sleep

If you do nothing else, try one or all of these tips for better sleep.

1. Get on Schedule For consistently deep and peaceful sleep, do everything you can to turn in at the same time every night, and wake up within an hour of the same time every day—even on weekends.

2. Cut Caffeine Everyone reacts to caffeine differently, but the general rule is this: No more than 250 milligrams a day—that's two to three cups of coffee—no later than 2 P.M. (Remember, if you start sleeping soundly, you won't need a pick-me-up!)

3. Exercise! Regular workouts (aim for 30 minutes at least three times a week) won't just tire you out on a daily basis; research shows they could lead to improved sleep over time.

4. Wind Down You can't slam on the brakes. Use the hour before bed to unplug from your computer and phone and relax your brain and body, so that they get the clear signal that it's time to sleep.

5. Prep Your Bedroom Make it cool (67°F to 70°F is ideal), dark (even the light from your phone or alarm clock display can wake you!) and quiet (earplugs or a white noise machine can cancel out snoring or traffic). This environment lulls you to sleep and keeps you there.

6. Have an Insomnia Strategy Sleepless nights will strike—the key is staying calm. Having a go-to distraction tactic (like counting backward by threes or getting out of bed to listen to soothing music) will help.

7. Speak Up! Don't keep sleep troubles to yourself or self-medicate past two weeks. Talk to your doctor so you can find the root cause and a lasting solution.

Stress Less

9

Simple ways to cope with your life— for ultimate health and happiness.

66 The most important thing is to enjoy your life— it's all that matters." *- Audrey Hepburn*

s it *possible* to be busier? Your schedule is taxing, and at times you think you're about to unravel. But everyone feels like that, right? "It's really easy to get on the bandwagon that life is meant to be stressful," says Susan Krauss Whitbourne, PhD, professor of psychology at the University of Massachusetts Amherst. "But you need to acknowledge that feeling like you're spread too thin on a regular basis is not healthy."

That's because—when you're stressed, anxious, angry, or all of the above—your body releases a hormone called cortisol, which is designed to help you face danger. Once in a while, that stress response can give you a healthy boost when you really need it (think: getting through a big presentation at work). But letting that cortisol build up in your bloodstream over time can wreak havoc on your mental and physical health. "Stress can wear out your body tissues. And emotionally, it impairs your ability to think clearly," says Alex Lickerman, MD, an expert in mind-body health and author of *The Undefeated Mind*.

Relieving stress—and replacing those stress hormones with happy brain chemicals—can have a host of benefits, which improve your health and help you look *and* feel younger. Among some of the most powerful:

- **You'll protect your heart.** Stress hormones raise your blood pressure and increase inflammation—two major risk factors for cardiovascular disease. (Relaxation, on the other hand, slows down your heart rate, for a healthier ticker.)

- **You'll lose belly fat.** Not only does stress affect your appetite and contribute to cravings, but it can actually cause you to pack on pounds around your middle, even if you're otherwise thin.

- **You'll save your skin.** Research shows that even minor stress affects the way your skin repairs itself, and subconscious muscle tension (a furrowed brow or clenched jaw) can lead to wrinkles.

- **You'll have more energy.** Learning to deal with your worry helps you sleep better and will stop the stress response that sends your body into overdrive.

How to use this chapter

We've divided the advice into two sections, which can help you overcome the mental traps that are holding you back from true satisfaction:

- **Reset Your Mindset** This section is about finding calm and improving your overall sense of satisfaction. Do you have trouble with work-life balance? Do wish you could ditch that vague sense of dread? These exercises and habit rehabs provide relaxation— and rewire your brain for more happiness in the long run, too.

- **Learn Quickie Mood Makeovers** Here you'll arm yourself with the in-the-moment coping mechanisms you need to prevent one little misstep or uncontrollable event (for instance, an angry email from your boss or a fight with your friend) from setting off the silent alarm system that hijacks your brain and derails your day.

MINI-MAKEOVER #1
Center Yourself Before You Get Out of Bed

A simple **2-minute meditation** (what's that? See: Ask the Experts, *below*) can relax you for the day ahead. After waking up, sit on the edge of your mattress for a moment (feet on the floor, back straight, and chin lifted) and follow these easy steps:

1 **Inhale deeply for four counts, then exhale for the same length of time.** Deep breathing triggers your body's relaxation response, slowing your heartbeat and lowering your blood pressure. Make sure the air coming in through your nose fully fills your lungs, and your lower belly rises.

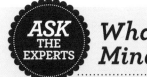

ASK THE EXPERTS *What are Meditation and Mindfulness?*

While these practices differ slightly, it's best to think of them both as mental breaks, says Jane Pernotto Ehrman, MEd, a behavioral specialist at the Cleveland Clinic's Center for Lifestyle Medicine. "We live in a culture of doing," she explains. "This is about just being. " By teaching your brain to be positive and present—while also showing your body true relaxation—you can eventually make "calm" your natural state. And in the meantime? You're acknowledging the source of your anxiety or temporarily removing yourself from the pressures of your day, which has an immediate effect on your stress levels.

2 **As you breathe in and out, focus on a positive thought.** Accept your life at this very moment, and practice self-compassion by replacing negative thoughts ("I'm going to fail") with something more upbeat ("I'm doing my best" or "This will all work out").

3 **Repeat for 2 minutes.** You'll start to feel calmer instantly, and combining positive self-talk and deep breathing daily can prevent thoughts from spiraling out of control, says Adam Burke, PhD, professor of health education and director for Holistic Health Studies, San Francisco State University.

This works especially well if: You often wake up with a sense of dread, or have trouble pulling yourself out of bed when facing a busy day ahead.

BONUS FASHION FIX
Dress for less stress

It seems almost silly—but what you wear *can* have an impact on how you feel on the inside.

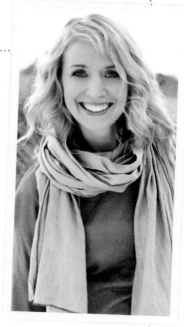

- **Sport something bright.** Just putting on one in a bold color can give you a lift, says Jennifer Baumgartner, PsyD, psychologist and author of *You Are What You Wear*. Shades of red, pink and yellow are best for stimulating your brain.

- **Put on fancy underwear.** In a *Consumer Reports* poll, almost 30 percent of women said that wearing unattractive or ill-fitting undies bums them out, while 47 percent said a special pair gives them a boost.

MINI-MAKEOVER #2
Mind the Mundane

Stress often takes on a life of its own, and here's why: Our minds are constantly in the past or the future—"we either ruminate on what we can't change or catastrophize about what hasn't happened yet," says Diana Winston, Ph.D., author of *Fully Present: The Science, Art, and Practice of Mindfulness*. But the more you practice coming back to the present (it's called mindfulness), the better you get at doing it. Her best tip: Turn a boring task you do daily into a mindfulness exercise. That way, you aren't just taking a short "time out" from your current anxiety; you're also learning what it feels like to snap yourself out of autopilot mode. So while washing the dishes, for example:

1 **Stop your thoughts.** As you do, start breathing deeply into your stomach, slowly and steadily, in and out.

2 **Focus on the physical sensations:** Feel the wetness and heat. Listen to the water run. This grounds you in the moment and helps to clear your mind.

Your mind may drift back to your worries or to-do list, but every time it does, follow these steps to bring your attention back to the moment. Tip: You can also do this as you're eating breakfast or lunch (in fact, chewing slowly and savoring the taste of your food is an excellent strategy to keep you from overeating too).

This works especially well if: Your mind always wanders to the worst-case scenario, you are plagued by guilt, or you feel so "crazy busy" you've been irritable or forgetful.

MINI-MAKEOVER #3
Meditate in Motion

Without a doubt, exercise is one of the most powerful mood improvers there is, and every single woman has it at her disposal. So if you're already walking or working out regularly, that's great! You're boosting your endorphins (the brain's feel-good chemicals) and relieving physical tension, both of which increase your energy and optimism. But there are ways to get even more bang for your buck, like this easy walking meditation from Nina Smiley, PhD, co-author of *The Three-Minute Meditator*—it'll quiet your mind while you move your body:

- **Where to do it:** Find a safe space to walk without traffic, like a park or sidewalk around your office building, or climb the stairs

QUICK TIP

Delegate. "Women confuse self-care with selfishness," says Pernotto Ehrman. But it's OK to have your teen do her laundry while you exercise. "Be the role model many of us didn't have—you're showing her that 'me time' is important too."

- **What it is:** You're essentially counting your steps and matching them to your breath:

  1. Deeply breathe in for four steps

  2. Deeply breathe out for four steps

  3. Repeat for at least 5 minutes

- **Why it relieves stress:** The breathing will relax your body, the counting will take your mind off your worries, and moving often wakes up your brain, which triggers creative solutions to your problems. It's great any time, but if you squeeze it in on your lunch or work break, it'll also give you a boost in productivity when you return to your desk.

This works especially well if: You don't otherwise exercise, or you need a quick break from work stress.

HABIT REHAB
Stop Slumping

Believe it or not, the way you sit can make you feel more stressed. So build in posture checks throughout the day by setting an hourly alert on your phone or computer. When you hear it ding, follow these simple steps:

- Chin up

- Shoulders down

- Feet flat on floor

Proper posture will naturally expand your chest so you take in more oxygen, which in turn helps calm your body's physical and emotional response to stress.

MINI-MAKEOVER #4
Do a Daily Download

Whatever stress and pressure you're feeling, it's important to get it out. For many women, it helps to talk to a friend or partner. Others, however, feel they benefit more from taking that mental clutter and putting it down on paper. For one, there's zero risk of judgment—plus you sidestep a common danger: talking your problems in circles. (That's no better than fixating on them yourself.) This simple 5-minute mind-dump routine can clear a toxic stress block-up, and it will also help you overcome negative thinking. Just create a document on your computer and:

Minute 1: Dump Spill the contents of your brain, no holds barred. You're basically focusing in on the background chitchat that's always there, then typing it out stream-of-consciousness style:

- I can't believe I didn't call the plumber. I'm such an idiot!

- I hate it when I miss the gym in the morning. I feel so blah. I really wish I went.

- My boss keeps bragging about his expensive vacation and I'm going nuts!

- Why hasn't Karen replied to my email from yesterday? Is she mad at me?

Minute 2: Evaluate Read what you wrote, and immediately wipe out any worries or thoughts that aren't in your control. You'd be surprised— the mere act of hitting delete helps you let these energy zappers go.

Minutes 3 to 4: Reframe Now, push yourself to change the conversation.

Take the stuff that's bugging you, and recast it in a hopeful manner:

- I'll write a note to call the plumber first thing tomorrow morning.

- I didn't make it to the gym, but I can still walk for 10 minutes after dinner.

- My friend might just be busy! I should resend again—or let it go.

Minute 5: Breathe Check your posture (See: Habit Rehab, p. 302), then close your eyes and breathe slowly and deeply (in-2-3-4, out-2-3-4). Then, get on with your day—calmer and more relaxed!

This works especially well if: Stress has been clouding your ability to focus or think clearly, or you struggle with a vague sense of worry that keeps you up at night (in that case, do this exercise before bed).

MINI-MAKEOVER #5
Create Clear Boundaries

You're probably juggling an incredible amount of responsibility, and if you're letting job stress seep into your family life (and vice versa), you're not alone. "For many women, there's still this expectation that they need to do it all—and do it all really well," says Dr. Lickerman. While there's no way to completely separate your dual duties, this work-life balance strategy can help you transition smoothly from one role to the next.

1 **Put up a wall.** Telling your boss, supervisor or direct reports "here's when I'm available again" can create mental closure before you go home. And in the opposite direction, setting up a solid time to check in with your kids or husband during the day limits your distractions, so you can focus fully on work.

2 Turn "to-do" into "it's done." Writing down what you need to do the next day gives you control over your workload before you leave the office, but it can also make you feel tired instead of inspired. So, once you're done, also jot down 10 quick things you've accomplished today or this week. This will give you a sense of achievement that quiets the worry and sends you home smiling.

3 Take a moment to acknowledge the transition. When you know you have to deal with a whole different set of stressors, use this "bodyscan" technique from Dr. Smiley, which relieves muscle tension and mental stress. Just sit in your car for 1 minute before going into work (in the morning) or your house (at the end of the day) and:

- Start by clenching your eyes and forehead for a moment, then let it go.

- As you release the tension, breathe out, warm and heavy.

- Work your way down, doing this with different body parts (jaw, chest, hands, etc.) all the way to your toes.

This works especially well if: You struggle with work-life balance or "my to-do list is never done!" anxiety.

Create a Stress-Less Sanctuary at Work

Follow this research-proven, expert-approved advice so your surroundings—whether you toil away in an office, classroom, cube or the corner of your living room—relax and inspire you:

1. Give your desk life. Something as simple as adding a plant or flowers won't just reduce stress, it can boost workplace productivity and increase your ability to come up with creative solutions, according to a Texas A&M study.

2. Tack up three photos. You don't even have to display them, but having a few strategic pictures on hand can soothe you in times of worry or doubt. Choose one that takes you to a happy place (like a beach sunset from your honeymoon); one of the "team" of family and friends that will always have your back; and one that boosts your confidence by reminding you of a major accomplishment (for instance, a snapshot from the first 5K you finished).

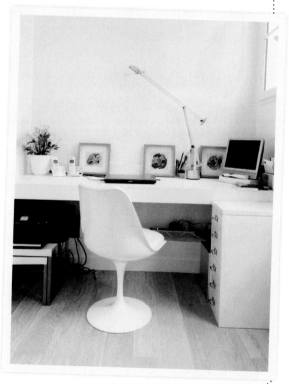

3. Clean up clutter. Clearing your desk can clear your mind, because clutter sends a sneaky signal to your brain that your work is never done. So even if you do nothing else, take 10 minutes every Friday afternoon to file what you need, toss what you don't and organize your supplies. You'll leave for the weekend feeling more in control—and start your new week more refreshed.

MINI-MAKEOVER #6
Take Time Out to Say "Thanks"

QUICK TIP
Download this app.
Gratitude Journal 365 (free, iTunes) helps you create a daily list of thanks and illustrate entries with personal photos.

Studies show that the regular practice of gratitude won't just make you happier—it can also yield major benefits, ranging from fewer doctor visits to lower heart-disease risk. But giving thanks needs to be a daily habit. Here, five different ways to tap the power:

1 **Collect Your Reflections** Keep a gratitude journal on your night-stand and write down what you're thankful for at the end of each day. As you fill it up, you'll have a physical reminder of your blessings, and over time, your outlook will shift too. (Searching for the positive after a rough day teaches you to be more optimistic.) To be sure your entry carries weight, make it as specific as possible. Writing one paragraph on how your husband was able to make you laugh in the midst of today's mini-crisis, for example, will be more beneficial than creating a laundry list of universal blessings, like family, health and a roof over your head.

2 **Say Grace Before a Meal** The simple ritual of expressing deep gratitude for the food you're about to eat makes you feel lucky to have it, and it can actually help you eat *better* too. How? By pausing to say a few words first, you're forced to slow down and direct your senses to the dish in front of you, which quells mindless munching.

3 **Share a Happy Status Update** To more deeply appreciate a small but significant event that comes your way, like a gorgeous sunset, post about it on a public forum like Twitter or Facebook. By typing

STRESS LESS

QUICK TIP

Urge to splurge?
Before you soothe yourself with retail therapy, know this: Research shows that spending on experiences (like a vacation with your family) rather than material things (a fancier car or a new pair of shoes) boosts bliss more. Why? Probably because you keep replaying the positive memories—and feel a lasting connection to the people you share them with.

out a quick sentence and hitting send, you're stopping for long enough to acknowledge your good fortune *and* you're sharing that gratitude with others, which helps you feel connected.

4 **Refocus Your Fitness** If you view workouts as burdens and not blessings, think about the gifts that something as simple as walking for 20 minutes can give you, like a stronger body, a reduced risk of disease and a longer life. You'll be more motivated to work out, and once you do, you'll have plenty of time to contemplate your *other* blessings. (Proof that it works: Research indicates that those who routinely expressed gratitude exercised 33 percent more per week and had more body confidence than those who weren't thankful.)

5 **Write a Note** Several studies show that writing a gratitude letter to someone who has been kind to you—even if you don't actually send it—leads to a boost in happiness. So pull out a sheet of stationary and thank someone from your past, whether it's the high school teacher who encouraged you to apply to college or the nurse who cared for your dad at the very end.

This works especially well if: You wish you could be more positive or are feeling down about certain life circumstances, like your weight, your job or your financial situation.

Easy Ways to Deal

Stress "isn't the bad things that happen to you or what you have on your plate—those are facts of life," says Dr. Lickerman. "What it really comes down to is, how equipped are you to handle them?" The Mini-Makeovers on the pages that follow will arm you with the coping tactics you need to outsmart stress and quiet negative thoughts in specific situations. With these targeted tools in your back pocket, you can snap yourself out of the stress response, so that one little misstep or unfortunate event doesn't derail your entire day.

MINI-MAKEOVER #7
End "Panic Mode"

When you're trying to calm down, deep breathing should be your go-to strategy. "By forcing yourself to breathe as you do in your most relaxed moments, you trick your body into releasing calming neurohormones, causing a biological shift in how you feel," says psychotherapist Belleruth Naparstek. "Just inhale and feel your abdomen expand. Go as slowly as possible, counting in—1-2-3. Then, observe the turn of your breath, and breathe it out—1-2-3. Whether you do this for 1 minute or 5, it's going to bring you to a calmer place."

This works especially well if: You get a phone call with bad news.

MINI-MAKEOVER #8
Get Over a Mistake

The best way to bounce back is to stop obsessing over it and find another focus right away. According to research from Ohio University, shifting gears mentally will stop your body's stress response and improve your mood. Thoroughly distracting yourself works best, so give yourself a specific task that you can do for 5 minutes (and that will put you in a concentration zone!), like working on a crossword puzzle.

This works especially well if: You goof up at work.

MINI-MAKEOVER #9:
Calm a Hot Head

When anger runs deep, channeling your frustration into physical tension might help too, says Pernotto Ehrman. As you inhale, clench your fists under the table, tighten your jaw, and squeeze every muscle. Then, as you exhale, let your body go loose, and...release.

This works especially well if: You get an obnoxious email from a colleague or your husband forgets to pick up the milk on his way home.

How Do I Stop Eating Junk When I'm Upset?

"The key is to distract yourself and channel your frustration or anxiety into something other than food," says Joy Bauer, RD. Before you eat: Squeeze a stress ball for 5 minutes, do 25 jumping jacks, then nurse a mug of hot tea. Post this plan front and center on your fridge to help you avoid eating the next time you're battling emotions or stress. Also keep a stash of healthy snack foods on hand: vegetables, like baby carrots, celery sticks, cucumber or bell pepper slices dipped in hummus or light ranch dressing, and fruit like apples or pears dipped in yogurt. The textures and crunch will satisfy your craving.

Pulling Through Tough Times

It's easy to feel thankful when everything is going your way. But what happens when you're hit with an unexpected challenge, like illness or grief? Gratitude can reenergize you during a crisis. When the chips are down:

1. Appreciate what you can control. You can't undo the past and may be unable to change your present circumstances. Instead, reframe your hardship to play up gratitude. Instead of beating yourself up for gaining weight, try: *I'm disappointed, but I'm thankful I can start fresh tomorrow.*

2. Picture a tougher break. In those moments when you can't see any silver lining, try to appreciate the ways in which you've been spared. For example, if your car was totaled while parked on a busy street, your first impulse might be to curse your bad luck. Instead, think: *Imagine how awful it would've been if I had been driving.* This simple strategy can reduce the "woe is me" feeling.

3. Draw from past difficulties. Reflect on your worst moments, your sorrows, your losses and your sadness. Then acknowledge that you are here, you are a survivor—and stronger for it too. This combination of grit and gratitude can help see you through.

MINI-MAKEOVER #10
Survive a Difficult Task

Let's say your boss gives you an impossible assignment at work, or you have to play nice with someone who grates on your nerves. Use "smile therapy"—because grinning and bearing it *really* works. One study found that people who smiled as they did difficult tasks (such as drawing with their non-dominant hand) had lower heart rates than people who kept a neutral expression.

This works especially well if: You're overwhelmed by a project or need to do something you dread.

MINI-MAKEOVER #11
Let Go of Anger or Disappointment

For a slight that's still bugging you hours (or days) later, do a simple vent whenever you notice the negative feelings pop up: Write down what's upsetting you, then throw out the paper. Researchers found that this activity can help you mentally release the thought and any lingering frustration. And no cheating! Throwing it out isn't enough if you only imagine doing so—study participants who physically tossed their notes into the trash benefitted most.

This works especially well if: You're disappointed in a friend or family member or fuming over a nasty comment from a friend.

MINI-MAKEOVER #12
Stop the Spiral of Worry

Talk to yourself. Research shows that repetition can help you calm down and keep your mind from running wild, says Lissa Rankin, MD, author of *Mind Over Medicine: Scientific Proof That You Can Heal Yourself.* So when you're overwhelmed, repeat a word, sound or phrase (like "everything is fine" or "relax") to yourself or out loud for at least 10 seconds. And if you still don't believe it? Think back and find a time when you tackled a task that was just as daunting, or survived a day just as busy. (So you can realistically say: "I've done it before. I can do it again.")

This works especially well if: You're staring at an endless to-do list or feel anxious about a busy day.

4 Little Ways to Find More Happiness

Additional quick tricks for working a meaningful mood boost into your day:

1. **Connect before bed.** One study found that levels of positive emotions in women peaked at 7 P.M. and lasted the rest of the night. Doing something social —whether it's calling your sister or watching TV with your son—maximizes these natural feelings of calm.

2. **Get crafty.** Research links being creative with feeling more content, but part of the lift you get is about taking time for you. When you go back to an old hobby like sewing or baking, you're reconnecting with your core identity—something that gets a little lost when you're busy caring for everyone else.

3. **Help a neighbor.** Doing a good deed—no matter how small—is a powerful de-stressor. It takes your mind off your problems and helps put them into perspective. Little actions—like carrying a neighbor's groceries—absolutely count. You can also seek out bigger volunteer opportunities at *volunteermatch.org*.

4. **Practice random acts of hugging.** Research shows that women whose partners hug them more have higher levels of oxytocin (a.k.a. the "love hormone") and lower blood pressure. Walking arm in arm with a loved one or petting an animal can also have the same effect.

MINI-MAKEOVER #13
Boost Your Confidence

When nerves or self-doubt creep in, it helps to do something called rehearsal imagery. You're simply walking yourself through what you're about to do and visualizing your best-case scenario. So if you have to give a speech? Duck into a bathroom stall, close your eyes and picture yourself delivering it flawlessly, followed by lots of applause and compliments. You can also rehearse difficult conversations—imagine yourself thinking on the spot and stand your ground will relieve your anxiety now, and give you a "been there, done that" sense of self-assurance.

This works especially well if: You need to speak in public or are facing a high-pressure conversation, like negotiating a raise.

3 More Ways to Relieve Stress (in 1 Minute or Less)

1. Reach for the sky. Get on your feet, look to the ceiling and stretch your arms straight up, spreading your fingers. "The simple act of standing prompts a boost in circulation, delivering oxygen and energy-rich blood to your cells," explains psychotherapist Kimberly Willis, PhD. And smile as you hold the stretch: It will trigger the release of feel-good brain chemicals.

2. Contact a friend. Your body releases oxytocin (a calming hormone) when you get in touch with a favorite friend or family member who you know will make you feel good. Connecting with a loved one through Facebook or email can have the same soothing effect as if you're speaking face-to-face.

3. Try acupressure. Rub an acupressure point that helps release tension in your body, suggests Dr. Willis. Grab the skin between your thumb and first finger with the thumb and first finger of your other hand. Gently massage in circles for 30 seconds, then repeat on the other hand.

The Quickie Guide to Stress Relief

If you do nothing else, try one or all of tips for more happiness.

1. Take a Break Refocusing your mindset daily is crucial, even if it's just a 2-minute meditation or a quick timeout to say "thanks." You'll stamp out short-term stress while retraining your brain to be calmer and more positive in the long term.

2. Move More! Exercise is quite possibly the most powerful stress reliever there is, plus it's available anytime and anywhere. So when in doubt, try walking away from your problems—literally. You'll gain clarity and boost endorphins.

3. Breathe...Deeply and Often Make sure the air coming in through your nose fully fills your lungs, so that your lower belly rises (in-2-3-4). Then, exhale slowly (out-2-3-4). This triggers a relaxation response throughout your entire body.

4. Be Here Now. Make this your mantra. The more you practice coming back to the present, the less time you'll spend fixating on your mistakes or worrying about the future.

5. Use Your "Team" Having close-knit people you can count on makes you feel unshakeable. Identify who they are for you (a friend, a sister, a colleague, your husband)—and ask for help in times of stress.

6. Set Boundaries Telling your boss you're unavailable over the weekend can help you leave work stress at the office. Likewise, asking your husband to only call you in an emergency while you're out for a walk will give you the "me time" you deserve.

7. Have an Emergency Action Plan Learning easy in-the-moment tactics to stop the stress response in its tracks will prevent tiny slipups from snowballing into larger-than-life disasters in your head.

Meet the 7 Years Younger Experts

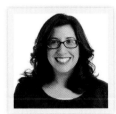

Annemarie Conte is the executive editor of *Woman's Day* magazine

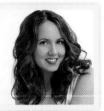

Melissa Matthews Brown is the beauty editor of *Woman's Day* magazine

Andrea Coombs Angrilla is a makeup artist with Laura Geller Beauty.

Robert T. Anolik, MD, is a dermatologist and clinical assistant professor |of dermatology at both the NYU School of Medicine and Weill Cornell Medical College of Cornell University. *robertanolikmd.com*

Birnur K. Aral, PhD, is the health, beauty & environmental sciences director at the Good Housekeeping Research Institute in New York City.

Donna Arand, PhD, is the clinical director of the Kettering Sleep Disorders Center in Dayton, OH.

Nick Arrojo is a celebrity hairstylist and owner of Arrojo Studio in New York City. *arrojonyc.com*

David E. Bank, MD, is a dermatologist and the director of The Center for Dermatology, Cosmetic & Laser Surgery in Mt. Kisco, New York. *thecenterforderm.com/ physicians/d_bank*

Joy Bauer, RD, is a registered dietitian in New York City, author of *Food Cures*, the nutrition and health expert for NBC's *TODAY* show, and a regular contributor to *Woman's Day* magazine. *joybauer.com*

Sasha Belousova is a hair removal expert at Paul Labrecque Salon and Spa in New York City. *paullabrecque.com*

Robin Berger is lead therapist at Cornelia Spa in New York City. *corneliaspaatthesurrey.com*

Diane Berson, MD, is an associate professor of dermatology at Weill Medical College of Cornell University and an assistant attending dermatologist at the New York-Presbyterian Hospital. *dianebersonmd.com*

Ramona Braganza is a celebrity trainer whose clients have included Jessica Alba, Halle Berry, Kate Beckinsale and Anne Hathaway. *ramonabraganza.com*

Michael Breus, PhD, is a clinical psychologist with a specialty in sleep disorders and the author of *The Sleep Doctor's Diet Plan. thesleepdoctor.com*

Stephanie Brown is a colorist at Nunzio Saviano Salon in New York City. *nunziosaviano.com/team*

Adam Burke, PhD, is professor of health education and director for Holistic Health Studies, San Francisco State University. *sfsu.edu/~ihhs/faculty.html*

Jenn Burke is Fitness Manager for Crunch Gyms in Los Angeles.

Valerie Callender, MD, is an associate professor of dermatology at Howard University College of Medicine in Washington, DC, and an expert in pigmentation disorders. *callenderskin.com*

Shirley Chi, MD, is a dermatologist at the Center for Advanced Dermatology in Arcadia, CA. *centerforadvanceddermatology.com*

Scott Collier, PhD, is director of the Vascular Biology and Autonomic Studies Laboratory at Appalachian State University. *hles.appstate.edu/scott-collier*

Nancy Collop, MD is director of the Emory Sleep Center and a past president of the American Academy of Sleep Medicine. *emoryhealthcare.org/physicians/c/collop-nancy*

Rodney Cutler is a celebrity hairstylist with salons located in New York City and Miami. *cutlersalon.com*

Doris Day, MD, is a New York City dermatologist, a clinical assistant professor of dermatology at the New York University Langone Medical Center, and author of *Forget the Facelift. myclearskin.com*

Landy Dean is a celebrity makeup artist and eyebrow expert. *landydean.com*

Aurora Dinu is a nail technician at Paul Labrecque Salon in New York City. *paullabrecque.com*

Amy Dixon is a personal trainer and the star of the *Motion Traxx: Treadmill Coach* audio workout. *amydixonfitness.com*

Jeanine Downie, MD, is the director of Image Dermatology in Montclair, NJ. *imagedermatology.com*

Donna Duarte-Ladd is the style editor at *Woman's Day* magazine

Pati Dubroff is a celebrity makeup artist who has worked with Gwyneth Paltrow, Jessica Biel and Eva Mendes. *patidubroff.com*

Lawrence Epstein, MD, is chief medical officer of the Sleep HealthCenters and an instructor at Harvard Medical School.

Susie Esther, MD, is a Charlotte-based sleep specialist and spokesperson for the American Academy of Sleep Medicine.

Barbara Fazio is a hairstylist and the owner of Cleveland's B. Fazio salon. *bfazio.com*

Taylor Fennema is a hairstylist at Oscar Blandi Salon in New York City.

Paul J. Frank, MD, is founder and director of The Fifth Avenue Dermatology Surgery and Laser Center in New York City. *pfrankmd.com*

Francesca Fusco, MD is a New York City dermatologist specializing in hair and scalp health. She practices at Wexler Dermatology and is an assistant clinical professor of dermatology at Mount Sinai Hospital. *wexlerdermatology.com/meet-our-experts/francesca-fusco*

Todd Galati is a cycling expert and the director of credentialing for the American Council on Exercise. *acefitness.org/fitness-professionals/fitness-expert.aspx?expert=Todd-Galati*

Toni Garcia-Jackson is a hairstylist in Wilmington, DE, and an educator for Mizani hair products. *tonigarcia-jackson.com*

Laura Geller is a pro makeup artist, owner of Laura Geller Makeup in New York City, and creator of Laura Geller Beauty, a line of cosmetics available at *laurageller.com*.

Jeanette Graf, MD, is an Assistant Clinical Professor of Dermatology at Mount Sinai Medical Center in New York City and the author of *Stop Aging, Start Living*. *askdrgraf.com*

Kathy Gromer, MD, is a sleep medicine specialist at the Minnesota Sleep Institute in Minneapolis. *minnsleep.com/staff*

Karyn Grossman, MD, is a dermatologist at Grossman Dermatology in Santa Monica, CA. *grossmandermatology.com*

Maureen Hagan is a physical therapist and fitness expert, as well as the vice president of operations for the GoodLife Fitness Clubs in Canada. *mohagan.com*

Taymour Hallal is a brow specialist at Paul Labrecque Salon and Spa in New York City. *paullabrecque.com*

Rita Hazan is a hairstylist, hair color expert and owner of Rita Hazan Salon in New York City. *ritahazan.com*

Nichola Joss is a beauty and skincare specialist and the Global Beauty Ambassador for London's Sanctuary Spa. *nicholajoss.com*

Sonia Kashuk is a celebrity makeup artist. Her makeup line is sold at Target stores nationwide. *soniakashuk.com*

David Kingsley, PhD, is a New York City trichologist who treats hair and scalp conditions, as well as the creator British Science Formulations products for thinning hair. *hairandscalp.com*

Kristin Kirkpatrick, MS, RD, LN, is a wellness manager at the Cleveland Clinic Wellness Institute. *my.clevelandclinic.org/wellness/default.aspx*

Susan Krauss Whitbourne, PhD, is a professor of psychology at the University of Massachusetts Amherst and author of *The Search for Fulfillment*. *psych.umass.edu/people/susanwhitbourne*

Emmanuel Layliev, DDS, is a cosmetic dentist at the New York Center for Cosmetic Dentistry in New York City. *nyccd.com/about-nyccd/dr-emanuel-layliev*

Kathryn Lee, RN, PhD, is professor and associate dean for research at the University of California San Francisco School of Nursing. *nursing.ucsf.edu/faculty/kathryn-lee*

Amy Lewis, MD, is cosmetic dermatologist in New York City and an assistant clinical professor of dermatology at Yale University School of Medicine. *amyblewismd.com*

Alex Lickerman, MD, is an expert in mind-body health and author of *The Undefeated Mind*. *alexlickerman.com*

Deborah Lippmann is a celebrity manicurist and the founder and creative director of Deborah Lippmann, a luxury beauty line. *deborahlippmann.com*

Roy Liu works with Laura Geller Beauty.

Kevin Mancuso is a trichologist and celebrity hairstylist who has worked with Sienna Miller, Anne Hathaway and Demi Moore. He is also the creative director for Nexxus Salon Hair Care. *kevinmancuso.com*

Michael Mantell is a senior consultant in behavioral psychology for the American Council on Exercise. *drmichaelmantell.com*

Kenneth Mark, MD, is a dermatologist with offices in New York City; Southampton, NY; East Hampton, NY, and Aspen, CO. He is also a clinical assistant professor in the department of dermatology at NYU Langone Medical Center. *kennethmarkmd.com*

Ellen Marmur, MD, is a dermatologist in New York City and author of *Simple Skin Beauty: Every Woman's Guide to a Lifetime of Healthy, Gorgeous Skin.* *marmurmedical.com*

Jessica Matthews is an exercise physiologist, an assistant professor of exercise science at Miramar College, and spokesperson for the American Council on Exercise.

Tina McIntosh is a hair extension and replacement artist at Shear Art Salon in Tampa, FL, and a national educator for Ultratess hair extensions.

Patrick Melville is a hairstylist and owner of Patrick Melville Salon in New York City. *patrickmelville.com*

Melanie Mills is an Emmy Award–winning makeup artist. She worked on ABC's *Dancing With the Stars* for five years and is the founder of GLEAM by Melanie Mills, a line of body makeup sold worldwide. *melaniemillsmakeup.com*

Kristi Molinaro is a group fitness instructor and creator of the 30/60/90 class. *306090fitness.com*

Belleruth Naparstek is a psychotherapist and pioneer in the field of guided imagery. *belleruthnaparstek.com*

David Nieman, DrPH, is a professor in Appalachian State University's Department of Health, Leisure and Exercise Science, as well as a spokesperson for the American College of Sports Medicine.

Meghan O'Brien, MD, is a clinical instructor of dermatology at Weill Cornell Medical Center in New York City and consulting dermatologist for Physicians Formula. *triparkderm.com/profile4*

Robert Oexman, DC, is the director of the Sleep to Live Institute in Joplin, MD. *sleeptoliveinstitute.com/about/stli-team*

Philip Pelusi is a hairstylist and CEO of Tela Beauty Organics by Philip Pelusi. *philippelusi.com*

Jane Pernotto Ehrman, MEd, is a behavioral specialist at the Cleveland Clinic's Center for Lifestyle Medicine. *imagesofwellness.com*

Sue Pike is a New York City makeup artist who works for Laura Mercier.

Jordy Poon is a celebrity makeup artist in New York City.

Meredith Poppler is a spokesperson for the International Health, Racquet and Sportsclub Association. *ihrsa.org/staff*

Sarah Potempa is a celebrity hairstylist and the creator of the Beachwaver rotating curling iron. *sarahpotempa.com*

Lissa Rankin, MD, is the author of *Mind Over Medicine: Scientific Proof That You Can Heal Yourself* and founder of the Whole Health Medicine Institute. *lissarankin.com*

Diane Renz, LPC, is a psychotherapist in Boulder, CO. *yourgatewaytohealing.com*

Rebecca Restrepo is a global makeup artist for Elizabeth Arden. *rebeccarestrepo.com*

Jet Rhys is a hairstylist with salons located in Solana Beach and Hillcrest, CA. *jetrhys.com*

Mally Roncal is a celebrity makeup artist who has worked with Jennifer Lopez, Rihanna and Beyoncé. She is also the founder and president of Mally Beauty, a line of makeup and beauty products sold on QVC and in select department stores. *mallybeauty.com*

Thomas Roth, PhD, director of the Henry Ford Sleep Disorders and Research Center in Detroit.

Leslie Sansone is a fitness expert and founder of the *Walk at Home* DVD Series. *walkathome.com*

Nunzio Saviano is a hairstylist and owner of Nunzio Saviano Salon in New York City. *nunziosaviano.com*

Joanna Schlip, is a celebrity makeup artist who consults for Physicians Formula and has worked with Christina Applegate, Eva Longoria and Laura Linney. *joannaschlip.com/bio*

Neal Schultz, MD, is a dermatologist in New York City. *nealschultzmd.com*

Ava Shamban, MD, is an assistant clinical professor of dermatology at UCLA-Geffen School of Medicine and the author of *Heal Your Skin. avamd.com*

Carol Shaw is a celebrity makeup artist and founder of Lorac Cosmetics. *carolshaw.la*

Lisa Shives, MD, is a Chicago-based sleep specialist at Northshore Sleep Medicine and medical expert for *SleepBetter.org.* *nssleep.com*

Tippi Shorter is a celebrity hairstylist who has worked with Alicia Keys, Rihanna, Lady Gaga and Jennifer Hudson. She is also Aveda's Global Artistic Director for textured hair. *tippishorter.com*

Irwin Smigel, DDS, is a cosmetic dentist in New York City and the inventor of Supersmile Professional Teeth Whitening and Oral Care products. *smigel.com*

Nina Smiley, PhD, is the co-author of *The Three-Minute Meditator.*

Jessica Smith is a certified personal trainer and creator of the *Walking for Weight Loss, Wellness & Energy* DVD. *jessicasmithtv.com*

Kimberly Snyder is a celebrity nutritionist and author of *The Beauty Detox Foods. kimberlysnyder.net*

Elizabeth Somer, RD, is a nutritionist and the author of *Eat Your Way to Happiness. elizabethsomer.com*

Erik St. Louis, MD is an associate professor of neurology at Mayo Clinic College of Medicine.
mayoclinic.org/biographies/st-louis-erik-k-m-d/bio-20055179

Elizabeth Tanzi, MD, is a dermatologist at the Washington Institute of Dermatologic Laser Surgery in Washington, DC.
skinlaser.com

Jeni Thomas, PhD, is a Senior Scientist at Proctor & Gamble, where she helps to develop new products.
pantene.com/en-us/experts/Pages/jeni-thomas-expert-bio

Lauren Thompson is a hairstylist with the Nunzio Saviano Salon.

Joanna Vargas is a celebrity facialist based in New York City and founder of the Joanna Vargas Salon and Skincare Collection. *joannavargas.com*

Sania Vucetaj is a brow expert and owner of Sania's Brow Bar in New York City. *saniasbrowbar.com*

Heidi Waldorf, MD, is a New York City dermatologist and an associate clinical professor of dermatology at Mount Sinai Hospital. *mountsinai.org/profiles/heidi-a-waldorf*

Andre Walker is a celebrity hairstylist who has styled Oprah Winfrey's hair for the past 25 years and the author of *Andre Talks Hair. andrewalkerhair.com*

Patricia Wexler, MD, is an associate clinical professor of dermatology at Mount Sinai School of Medicine. She practices at Wexler Dermatology in New York City. *wexlerdermatology.com/meet-our-experts/patricia-wexler*

John Whelan is color director at Nunzio Saviano Salon in New York City. *nunziosaviano.com/team*

Kyle White is the lead colorist at Oscar Blandi Salon in New York City. His loyal clients include Mariah Carey, Julianna Margulies and Tatum O'Neal. *oscarblandi.com/staff_detail.php?id=18*

Cindy Whitmarsh is a personal trainer and creator of the UFIT series of fitness DVDs. *cindywhitmarshfitness.com*

Kimberly Willis, PhD, is a psychotherapist and the author of *The Little Book of Diet Help.*

Ni'Kita Wilson is CEO and Director of Innovation at Catalyst Cosmetic Development, which develops products for skincare and beauty brands. She is also the founder of *Skinects.com*, a site that helps women find the right products for their skin type. *skinects.com*

Diana Winston, PhD, is the Director of Mindfulness Education at the UCLA Mindful Awareness Research Center and author of *Fully Present: The Science, Art, and Practice of Mindfulness.*
http://marc.ucla.edu/body.cfm?id=19

Joshua Zeichner, MD, is the director of cosmetic and clinical research in dermatology at Mount Sinai Hospital in New York City. *zeichnerdermatology.com*

Index

Photography Credits

Cover images: Getty; iStock.

Makeover shoots: Photography by Shannon Greer; Hair by Nunzio Saviano Salon and Oscar Blandi Salon; Makeup by Laura Geller Salon and Sue Pike for Laura Mercier; Wardrobe by Maria-Stefania Vavylopoulou.

p. 5: Michael Waring; Hair & Makeup by Nikki Wang.

p. 10: Shannon Greer. p. 18: Shutterstock.

p. 58: Getty. p. 92: Shannon Greer.

p. 122: Michael Williams.

p. 136: Shutterstock; Jeffrey Westbrook/ Studio D; Greg Marino/Studio D.

p. 148: Getty.

p. 182: Steve Giralt.

p. 188: Shutterstock.

p. 190: Shutterstock.

p. 192: Getty.

p. 196: Ben Goldstein/Studio D.

p. 197: Getty.

p. 200: Shutterstock.

p. 202: Getty.

p. 205: Getty (2).

p. 206: Getty.

p. 209: Getty.

p. 211: Bruno Crescia Photography/Getty.

p. 212: Joseph De Leo/Getty.

p. 215: Alamy; Shutterstock.

p. 217: Getty. p. 218: Getty.

p. 219: Getty.

p. 222: Kevin Summers/Getty.

p. 224: Getty.

p. 227: Shutterstock.

p. 230: Getty.

p. 236: Keith Lathrop.

p. 255: Michael Waring.

p. 256: Philip Friedman/Studio D; Shannon Greer.

p. 257: Perry Hagopian; Susan Pittard/ Studio D.

p. 258: Keith Lathrop.

p. 259: Keith Lathrop; Philip Friedman/ Studio D.

p. 260: Philip Friedman/Studio D; Keith Lathrop.

p. 261: Perry Hagopian; Michael Waring.

p. 262: Michael Waring; Shannon Greer.

p. 263: Perry Hagopian.

p. 264: Susan Pittard/Studio D.

p. 265: Susan Pittard/Studio D; Perry Hagopian.

p. 266: Ben Goldstein/Studio D; Philip Friedman/Studio D.

p. 268: Getty.

p. 274: Getty.

p. 277: Cavan Images/Getty. p. 279: Getty.

p. 280: Douglas Gibb/ Photoshot.

p. 283: Getty; Shutterstock.

p. 291: Getty.

p. 294: Jose Luis Pelaez/Getty.

p. 299: Kristiane Vey/ Jump Fotoagentur.

p. 306: Julien Fernandez/GAP Interiors.

p. 313: Kristin Duvall/Getty.

p. 316: Susan Pittard/Studio D; Keith Lathrop.

The information in this book is not meant to take the place of the advice of your doctor. Before embarking on a weight loss program, you are advised to seek your doctor's counsel to make sure that the weight loss plan you choose is right for your particular needs. Further, this book's mention of products made by various companies does not imply that those companies endorse this book.

Cover design by Jill Armus
Interior design by Andrea Brake Lukeman

Joy Bauer has kindly granted permission to use her recipes in this book: pages 187, 188, 189, 191, 193, 197, 201, 206, 209, 212, 215, 217, 221

ISBN 978-1-936297-72-6
Cataloging-in-Publication Data available from the Library of Congress

10 9 8 7 6 5 4 3 2 1

Published by Hearst Editions/Hearst Magazines
300 West 57th Street
New York, NY 10019

Woman's Day and 7 Years Younger are registered trademarks of Hearst Communications, Inc.

www.womansday.com

www.7yearsyounger.com

Distributed to the trade by Hachette Book Group

All US and Canadian orders:
Hachette Book Group
Order Department
Three Center Plaza
Boston, MA 02108
Call toll free: 1-800-759-0190
Fax toll free: 1-800-286-9471

For information regarding discounts to corporations, organizations, non-book retailers and wholesalers; mail order catalogs; and premiums, contact:
Special Markets Department
Hachette Book Group
237 Park Avenue
New York, NY 10017
Call toll free: 1-800-222-6747
Fax toll free: 1-800-222-6902

For all international orders:
Hachette Book Group
237 Park Avenue
New York, NY 10017
Tel: 212-364-1325
Fax: 800-364-0933
international@hbgusa.com

Printed in the USA